Tai Chi Ch'uan: The Technique of Power

TAI CHI CH'UAN

The
Technique
of
Power

TEM HORWITZ
SUSAN KIMMELMAN
with H. H. LUI

CHICAGO REVIEW PRESS

First Edition

First Printing 1976

Published by
Chicago Review Press, Incorporated
811 West Junior Terrace
Chicago, Illinois 60613

Chicago Review Press Books are distributed by
The Swallow Press Incorporated
811 West Junior Terrace
Chicago, Illinois 60613

ISBN 0-914090-49-6

Library of Congress Catalog Number 76-41613

Book design and typography by Claire J. Mahoney

*Is there such a thing as perfect happiness in the world
or isn't there? Is there some way to keep yourself alive
or isn't there? What to do, what to rely on, what to avoid,
what to stick by, what to follow, what to leave alone,
what to find happiness in, what to hate?*

Chuang Tzu

Contents

Contents

Acknowledgments

The illustrations that are used at the beginning of each chapter of this book come from *Chinese Folk Designs: A Collection of 300 Cut-Paper Designs Used for Embroidery*, by W. M. Hawley, Dover Publications. The designs are: Chapter I a Dragon, II the Phoenix, III a Lotus Charm, IV Ch'ang Wo fleeing to the moon, V a Butterfly, VI Lu Tung-pin one of the Eight Immortals, patron of barbers, slays dragons, checks evil, cures the sick, VII Landscape, VIII the T'ang Emperor Ming visiting the moon for pleasure, IX Han Hsiang-tzu one of the Eight Immortals, the patron of musicians, and X a fairy scattering flowers.

The selections from the *Tao Te Ching* included in this book are from *Tao Te Ching*, by Lao Tzu, translated by Gia-fu Feng and Jane English. Reprinted by permission of Alfred A. Knopf, Inc.

The selections from the writings of Chuang Tzu included in this book are from Burton Watson (translator): *The Complete Works of Chuang Tzu*, New York: Columbia University Press, 1968, by permission of the publisher.

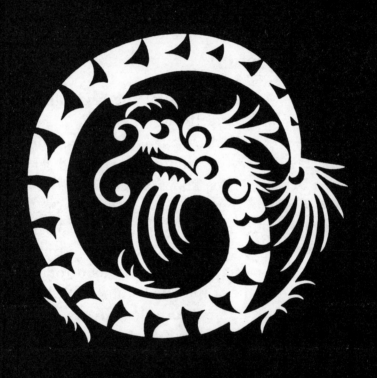

Preface and Dedication

This book is intended as an introduction and a reference. It is not possible to learn Tai Chi from a book, without a teacher. We have written in the hope of engaging your curiosity and offering inspiration to begin. For those already involved in Tai Chi we hope this will be a source book, opening the way to a study of the philosophy that gives meaning and substance to the exercise.

Our book is written for Westerners, by Westerners. Much of the Tai Chi literature to date falls into one of two categories. Books written by Orientals with an incomplete understanding of the Western perspective tend to be quaint and somewhat obscure, while books written in the effusive California flower style encourage unrealistic expectations. Tai Chi will not change your life in a week-end or in a week. It is a slow, slow process and you must be willing to be sometimes bored in order to learn the solace of repetition. Everyone yearns for inspiration. Tai Chi is genuine sustaining inspiration, but not of the lightning and thunder variety. The exercise gives its blessing in return for time and energy, and most of all patience.

We have written largely from our own experience. We are part of a collective of six that runs a dance-theatre and school in Chicago, where we perform and teach dance and Tai Chi. Our experience as part of this group is interwoven with our experience of Tai Chi for the last several years. In learning what sustains a collaboration, we are always struggling to free ourselves of pre-set definitions and expectations. We are grateful to the other members of the collective for their support both as generous friends and loyal adversaries.

Writing about something that you do gives a distance that brings clarity. Writing, we have learned the depth of our commitment and the strength of our faith. Tai Chi is at once precious and accessible to everyone, not just the young and hip and healthy. The exercise is a bridge between the cultures of East and West. Our teacher and guide across the bridge has been Hubert H. Lui. This book is dedicated, in endless gratitude, to him.

Tem Horwitz
Susan Kimmelman

Reflections on Getting Up in the Morning

Change. The central question of our collective and individual lives. We hunger for it desperately and resist it with an equal desperation. Everything changes too fast for us. We are overwhelmed by a world out of control. At the same time we are hopelessly impatient. Nothing ever seems to really change.

Change, says the dictionary,
> to cause to be different
> to give a different form or appearance to,
>> to transform
> to go from one phase to another, as the moon

What will sustain us? The style of change; the changing of style. Sustenance, not maintenance, is the human need. Sustenance implies the nourishment of living creatures, by a complex process daily changing food into flesh. Machines are maintained. To sustain ourselves we learn to change.

15

Tai Chi Ch'uan

Astrology, futurology, city-planning — we try to stay in control by predicting the patterns of change. We are growing every day more dissatisfied with the constant technological change (progress) that destroys the world as it makes life ever more convenient. This issue is now being discussed at great length, and not a moment too soon. Overwhelmed by a world seemingly beyond control, extraordinary numbers of people have begun to turn their energy to the search for inner change. Personal growth has become the watchword of a new and fervent faith. It is called the "human potential movement" and boasts a bewildering array of new and old techniques of physical, psychological and spiritual therapies. They all appeal to the same intense hunger, as contagious as the plague, a hunger to change, to grow, to be, finally, satisfied. What was it that Dick Diver wanted?

> He used to think that he wanted to be good, he wanted to be kind, he wanted to be brave and wise, but it was all pretty difficult. He wanted to be loved too, if he could fit it in.

It is tempting to criticize the thing wholesale, and to summarily dismiss the people who preach and practice these new religions. But there are so damn many, and they tell you that each new one is *it*, always better than what went before. The sheer variety of answers is a testimony to the unfulfilled desperation of the search. So we try one thing and then another in an endless attempt to establish both a grounded center and a free flow. Too often it seems that all we manage to do is swing wildly back and forth like pendulums gone berserk.

In the last gubernatorial election in this state, one of the candidates, the winning one, reportedly ate exactly the same lunch every day in order not to waste any time making unnecessary decisions. Many of my generation, carefully trained for efficiency (although perhaps not to that extreme) find upon reaching adulthood that all sense of direction suddenly and inexplicably has disappeared. I am talking about people whose lives are mapped out for them when they are children, from education to higher education to professional school, to profession and so on, from one success to another. When the pre-ordained pattern is broken in an effort to re-assert the self, the immediate reaction is often aimlessness. Follow anything to its extreme and you will find its opposite. Many of the most intelligent and talented people I knew in school spent a large share of their college years and beyond sitting in front of the TV screen.

Daily the pendulum swings in shorter arcs. We can recognize the extremes both of rigidity and of chaos in our lives from one day to the next. On Monday you come home from a meeting feeling like a fool because you've been so bull-headed and stubborn. The next day you're a jelly fish; from conversation to conversation you change your opinion until you no longer know what you think, or even if you think at all.

17

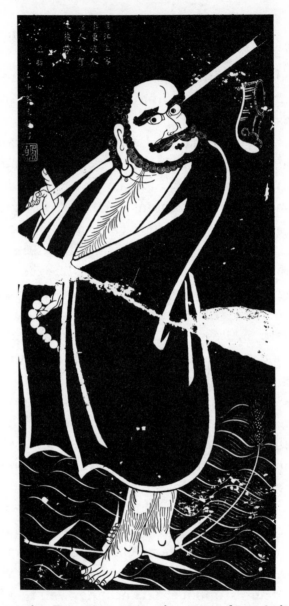

Bodhidharma, by Ting Yun-peng, who came from India to China preaching a kind of Buddhism which ultimately evolved into Ch'an or Zen Buddhism.
Courtesy of Field Museum of Natural History, Chicago.

Looking for a way out of the morass, a way to endure with some grace and compassion, many have recently turned to the philosophies of the Orient. We are concerned here most directly with Taoism. Every Westerner who writes about Taoism makes apologetic reference to the contradiction of trying to explain the inexplicable. The *Tao Te Ching*, the primary text of Taoism, begins like this: "The Tao that can be spoken of is not the true Tao." Writers usually go on to explain in various ways that to follow the Tao is to accept what is, to take one's part in the general flow and interdependence of the universe. It is an all-inclusive concept. By definition there is nothing outside of it — even if you resist it, your resistance is part of it, part of what is happening, and what is happening is what must happen. The central image is the circle, and the process by which each thing becomes its opposite. The unity of being contains within itself indissoluble oppositions. It is a philosophy of polarities in balance, not one of embattled contradictions. There is no coin with only one side, although often we can only see one side at a time.

Although it has become fashionable of late to denigrate Western science (mistaking the thing itself for our own unintelligent use of it), it is here that West echoes East. In the rarified air of higher mathematics and relativity theory the circle comes around again, or so we are told. Those of us with more basic scientific educations only have to recall the Laws of Motion that we copied down on the fresh white pages of our notebooks in eighth

19

grade: "Any action produces an opposite and equal re-action."

As a metaphor of our social and emotional lives this principle is a cliché. Clichés are a curious phenomenon — truths universally evident, and yet cheapened by constant repetition and simplification until they lose the substance of their meaning. This has been the sad fate, within the last few decades, of much of the Oriental philosophy that has found its way Westward. Who has not seen the poster or greeting card with a few well-chosen words from Lao Tzu concerning change and the cycles of the Universe, etc., etc.? A small clear bell of recognition rings the first time you see it and then it fades away in the over-abundance of words and pictures and hip decorating motifs.

For middle-class Americans who sense themselves caught up in an endless struggle for future satisfaction that recedes steadily as we approach it, Eastern thought has an obvious appeal. Unhappily for us, the hope of this new possibility has been largely dissipated. Every new idea becomes something to sell. The media, with its incredible power to popularize, manages at the same time to dilute and corrupt almost everything it touches.

Is there a way for us to honestly absorb this wisdom into *our* lives and cross this widest of cultural chasms between East and West? "What it has taken China thousands of years to build cannot be grasped by theft. We must instead earn it in order to possess it" (Jung). We can fill the bookcases with Alan Watts and translations of Lao Tzu, but where do we find the living spirit of the thought? Dutiful students, what do we do when we've read all the books and the questions persist? How do we make the knowledge live?

We learn with our bodies.

Change is motion.

Tai Chi is motion; change in motion. Moving and changing from up to down, from hard to soft, from in to out. Starting from the center, following the out-going energy until it folds back upon itself, always returning to center.

A profoundly physical experience, Tai Chi gives substance to the pretty words and catchy phrases. For the body allows no short-cuts and no pretenses. In the realm of the physical, enthusiasm is no substitute for persistence. Change happens slowly, through countless mornings and evenings. The gift is in proportion to one's initial commitment and persistent devotion. Day after day, no matter how inspiring the teacher, only you can make the commitment and exercise the devotion.

Our teacher, H. H. Lui, is fond of explaining how there is really no mystery to many apparently magical physical feats. He calls them "miscellaneous talents". "Do you want to learn Iron Fist?" he asks. "Go home for one hundred days and practice punching a bag for two hours each morning and night." His point is that there are just not many people willing to do that (and in fact he questions the value of using all that energy to perfect such an overly specialized 'art'.) The "secret" is sheer persistence.

It is this grounding of the "clichés" of self realization

in a sustained physical experience that has made me value Tai Chi above many of the other current possibilities for "self-improvement". After all, it is not enough to have one or two or several *peak* experiences and to be, the next day, a "changed" person. What we are after is to become "changing" people. Even the man who founded the Esalen Institute, who ought to know, if anyone does, about change and human potential techniques, has said as much:

> The hunger for this sort of thing is simply enormous and the risks are worth taking. But to run an encounter group for nine months is just not the answer. Esalen has been great for these openings up exercises but not for the long haul. The problem is to find sustaining ways of life, sustaining disciplines . . . You can't live on encounter.
>
>

The New Yorker, an article about Michael
Murphy by Calvin Trilling

Although there *are* people who teach week-end workshops in Tai Chi, claiming to communicate the quality of the movement without the burden of the form, this is in contradiction to the best of the Tai Chi experience. The discipline is indispensable. Tai Chi's unique strength lies in this integration of form and freedom.

This is the gift of Tai Chi. For it is very well to be organic and free-flowing, but how many of us can (or want) to wake up singing with the birds and to wander through the woods day after day? There are still decisions to be made, choices to be chosen, and work to be done. Freud, in disrepute these days, did remind us that honest work can be as nourishing as love. Taoism is more than a sophisticated justification for personal and social inertia. It does not dispense cheerfully with all organized activity and serious effort. The universe is seen as a cosmic organic flow of ever-changing patterns. Everything fits, but everything is not the same. And we are responsible for the patterns of our lives, of our days, of our art. The order is there; it must be discovered. This is the Tao. Jumping up and down and laughing with cosmic glee is only part of it. We learn to move gracefully through the changes of our lives by understanding and submitting ourselves to the forms, to the structures. When the structures are inadequate or unjust they must be reshaped. The form of life, or work, or family, new forms or old.

Tai Chi is form, moving through cycles of change, over and over again, gently and with freedom, carrying us through to the spirit within.

On the rebound from the work ethic we are ever ready to throw out all the babies with the gallons of dirty bath water. So we call an end, forever, to tedium and repetition. But an essential part of physical learning is the unconscious factor, which depends upon a kind of repetitious patterning. Watch the baby learn to walk, or ask any athlete or craftsman. The complexity of our physical mechanism is well known to exceed by far the limits of our conscious attention. Any one who has learned to do

23

anything physical well learns it in muscle and sinew and neural pathway, until it can be done, as we say, "blind-folded". So too with the lessons of Tai Chi as it re-teaches us balance and stillness and easy flow of motion.

Everyone has heard from friends and acquaintances frequent laments about lack of physical fitness. Over and over we say, "I have just got to do something to get into shape, got to get into something physical." But it is clear that most of the activities available for this purpose are difficult to sustain over time. The Canadian Air Force exercises for a few weeks, a few dance classes, a few push-ups. How *do* you bring disciplines into your life, if you haven't got the ambitions or motivation of a professional athlete or performer.

Discipline is oppressive when it is perceived as such. It becomes a constant struggle to do something which you do not want to do, but believe to be "good for you". Or a constant struggle not to do, or eat, or drink, things you feel you "want". Perhaps there is no satisfying answer to the question of how we come to desire that which makes us unhealthy. We know we are not hungry, and yet we want. Henderson the Rain King was tormented by a small plaintive voice from within. Every afternoon the voice said, "I want, I want, I want". But it never said what. Perhaps it is only human — this sense of an emptiness that is never filled. But if we are doomed to walk forever forward towards the carrot that dangles before our eyes, our liberation must be in our ability to accept, to understand, to be conscious.

The practice of Tai Chi is one way towards a resolution. In the beginning you practice because you have made a decision to do so. What begins as an exercise of will becomes by degrees less and less an externally imposed chore ("Now I am doing my exercises") and more and more a source of inner strength and a natural part of every day.

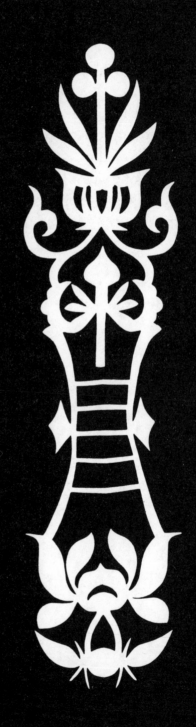

Tai Chi Ch'uan: The Power of Technique

For those readers who are complete strangers to Tai Chi, a basic description is in order. What is it?

Out of the great void, all things are generated by the interplay of positive and negative forces. The term Tai Chi, sometimes translated as "Supreme Ultimate", refers to this primal inter-action. Tai Chi also names the Yin-Yang symbol, designed in the eleventh century by a Sung metaphysician. This symbol, more and more familiar in the Western world, pictures an inviolable duality. The light and dark sides represent the two basic forces in the universe. The two sides are indissolubly connected by a smaller circle in the center of each representing its opposite. Circles within circles. Ch'uan means boxing, or fist, and is used to mean form, or kind of exercise. Tai Chi Ch'uan, supreme ultimate boxing, has also been called Mien Ch'uan, Cotton Fist, and Chan Ch'uan, Long Boxing, after the Yang Tze, or Long River. The movement is characterized by soft-

27

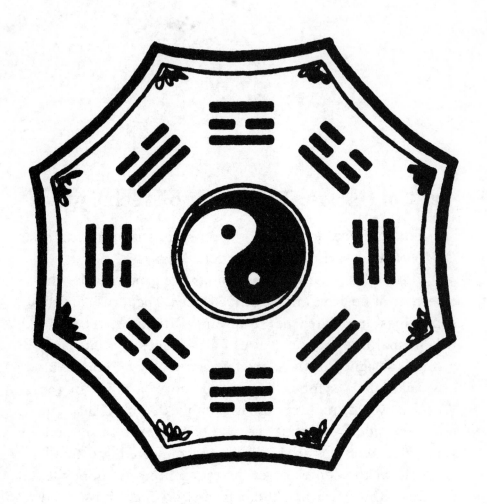

Tai Chi is the Supreme Ultimate likened to the ridge-pole of a house, the support on which every part of the building depends. In this illustration it is surrounded by the eight trigrams.

28

ness and a yielding quality, hence Cotton Fist, and by a continuous flowing of energy, like the waters of the Long River. The play of oppositions expressed by the Tai Chi symbol is symbolized kinetically in the exercise. Every movement is circular and out of each motion comes its opposite. You sink down before you stretch up; pull back before reaching out; shift left in order to swing right. The principles of Tai Chi are similar to the principles of those martial arts which emphasize self-defense. However, the exercise is also practiced alone for purposes of health and meditation.

The "form" is a precisely choreographed sequence of motion, anywhere from five to sixty minutes long, depending on which one you learn. Tai Chi is "played" in slow motion and is accompanied by deep and regular breathing. Each motion is co-ordinated with the breath: breathe out to sink down, breathe in to rise up; breathe out to deliver strength, breathe in to pull back.

At first the most difficult aspect of learning Tai Chi is memorizing the sequence, especially for adults who do not have much experience with this kind of motion memory. The form is absolutely specific with reference to direction and the shape and placement of each part of the body. It requires daily practice; the body learns only by doing. At some point (different for each learner) the vocabulary becomes familiar and natural, and the learning is much easier after that. Although difficult, this kind of learning is an essential part of the experience. The student is motivated to continue — you are clearly learning *something*. You must remember each motion, each direction, accumulating from week to week. There is the small thrill of increasing competence.

It can take a year or two to learn the sequence well enough so that it can be done without thinking constantly about what comes next. But once learned, the continuity has a clear advantage over more conventional exercises where you must stop and start, and stop and start again. The constant repetition of the form leads paradoxically to freedom. Body and mind, at least for a little while, are one.

Besides the learning of the form, most classes include various exercises to help in mastering the specific techniques of movement. Styles differ from form to form but the same basic principles can be recognized in every legitimate version. These principles correspond closely to the philosophical tenets of Taoism. Flexibility of the body is one way towards greater mental and emotional resilience. There are exercises for stretching the muscles and loosening the joints, particularly shoulders, which accumulate great tension in the course of our sedentary lives. This makes Tai Chi a help with circulatory problems and pre-arthritic conditions. Other basic exercises focus on balance — throughout the form the weight of the body shifts constantly from leg to leg. One foot always carries more than half the weight. "Double-weightedness", or standing with the weight equally distributed between both feet, is a grievous error because it limits agility. On another level, the lesson is to focus and to go deeper, avoiding the dissipation of energy in all directions at once: integrity of purpose as opposed to fragmentation.

Unlike Yoga, in Tai Chi the body is always upright. The skeleton hangs as though suspended from the crown of the head, relaxed through all the joints, so that the weight of the body sinks downward through the legs and feet. "Sinking the weight" establishes roots; the body re-learns its connection to the earth and eventually falls into a natural and relaxed posture. Tai Chi begins in stillness. It is a physical embodiment of the principle of "wu-wei", non-doing, non-acting. The movement originates and is generated from this stillness. On a practical level this is to say that the movement originates not with muscular force, but with an internal energy which is the product of breathing and thought. To experience this, stand with your feet together, shoulders dropped, arms hanging at your sides, knees slightly bent. Close your eyes and for a minute or two just concentrate on your breathing, letting it slow down and deepen. Try to imagine the air filling up your whole body, all the way down to your finger tips. With each inhalation try to feel the air floating your hands and arms out from the sides of your body. These small movements are Tai Chi. They grow from the inside out, they are effortless, and they differ radically from the motion of our everyday lives. Above all, the movements come from not-doing, from letting go. From the beginning stillness comes motion, always slow but never monotonous, rising and falling with a natural rhythm like the ocean.

At the beginning the student must concentrate on getting the movements perfectly smooth, with no gaps in the flow of energy. Later the movement takes on a life of its own, a gentle ebb and swell. One way of practicing is to repeat one small circular motion over and over again. This results in a kind of patterning — the body discovers its natural strength as the flow of energy establishes its pathway. Finally, it becomes automatic. On a crowded street someone pushes you, and instead of stiffening to resist, you yield easily, turning at the waist, completing the circles, free from the accumulation of muscular tension.

Traditionally, Tai Chi is taught with no verbal explanation; you merely follow the teacher. This method is not effective for Western students, who require some cultural translation. At its best, Tai Chi is filled with an internal vitality. The form is empty; the spirit makes it live. To unite the body and the mind, you must learn to think the motion and to move the thought. A good teacher can provide verbal and visual images to help in this integration of consciousness. An example. Standing solidly on two feet, with your knees slightly bent, raise your arms slowly straight in front of you to shoulder height. Lower them just as slowly. Breathe in as you raise the arms, and out as you lower them. Repeat this over and over, using no force to raise the arms, but "willing" them upward. Imagine as you do it that the air is thick, and viscous, like water. After a while, it will feel like the arms float up and down by themselves, with a peculiar light-heaviness. The body is swimming in the air. The fingers are heavy and tingle with the circulation of blood. The flesh is becoming conscious.

Tai Chi class as such is an experience in a very particular kind of sharing. Basically, the exercise is solitary and meditative. But practicing together week after week a group of students learns unconsciously to share internal energies. The impulses of motion are almost palpable — it looks as if everyone is being gently swept along by a single current. The class has a special ambience — polite and relaxed at the same time. In the modern zeal to banish repression forever, it begins to seem that the only legitimate group experience must be one of intense conflict. Tai Chi class demonstrates another possibility. Energy is shared, but boundaries are not violated. When fighting is not part of the training, the classroom situation is completely non-competitive; there is no standard of achievement. Only the individual can measure his or her growing peace and satisfaction. This is not to say that some people are not "better" at it than others. Everyone is *not* equal in potential. With persistence each one can develop to the limit of this given potential, and perhaps beyond. The eye learns gradually to distinguish the invisible in the visible, and to judge the quality of the motion. After a while you can "see" whether or not the energy is continuous and centered. But because everyone moves together, and concentrates so intensely, the normal self-consciousness is minimized and soon conquered.

Everyone learns at a different pace, and no one will look exactly the same. This is a constant source of reassurance and delight to us. Practicing an exercise called Cloud Hands, students close their eyes and move their arms in circles, swinging from the waist. After some time the movements lose their jerky, erratic quality, as each body finds its own rhythm and design. And each one is utterly different from the next. After the initial awkwardness is overcome, and the form is memorized, students continue to learn from one another's unique senses of motion. This uniqueness is a comfort to remember when crushed on crowded subways or humiliated by computers.

But the class is not enough. Like anything else, in order to get the most out of Tai Chi you have to make it your own. Practically, this means arranging your life so that you can and do practice every day, by yourself. Some teachers claim that ten minutes of daily practice is sufficient. This is false advertising. Tai Chi is not a magic panacea or any kind of instant short-cut. It's a fair deal — you receive in proportion to what you give.

The issue of discipline, central to Tai Chi, is a problematic one. Popular psychology has encouraged us to liberate ourselves from our compulsions and the attendant guilt and anxiety. But this liberation is a mixed blessing, at best. Perhaps self-discipline is a *healthy* compulsion. Who knows just where the line can be drawn? It's a curious paradox, but a common experience; most people find a modicum of structure a necessity. It is the form of our days that makes the empty spaces possible. Tai Chi can be an excellent source of this freedom-giving form.

You can practice in the morning, or in the evening, or both, for half an hour, or an hour, or more. You need very little space, and no special clothing or equipment.

The hardest step is the first, and you must take that first step many times. You begin with determination; you decide that you want to make this new thing a part of your life. Initially, it is an act of faith. So you try, and you find it's harder than you thought it would be to get up a little earlier. Maybe you manage to practice one day out of four. You must be patient, as well as persistent. Guilt is no help to this discipline. Instead of feeling frustrated by your expectations and giving up, you shrug and try tomorrow. When practicing becomes an empty task, it is necessary to lay back for a while in order to rediscover your own motivation. The discipline of the will requires the same paradoxical balance as the discipline of the body — absolute relaxation and absolute attention. Many people start Tai Chi and give it up, sometimes several times, before the time is right for them.

Eventually the persistence pays off. It grows on you and the effort becomes ease. You begin to look forward to that quiet, solitary hour. It is an empty time, as different each day as the weather. For people whose lives are crowded with activity it is permission to be quiet. For people who slide towards inertia, it is a way to set yourself in motion. In time, it becomes a dependable comfort and a part of the "dailiness of life". The inner quiet refreshes weary, overloaded senses. After practice the colors of familiar things have a new clarity. You learn that you *can* refuse to be interrupted. You don't have to answer the phone, just because it rings. Hopefully, eventually, you become able to accept the interruptions and irritations with genuine equanimity.

Expectations often make the difference between disappointment and satisfaction. It is a great disservice to Tai Chi to claim that it is an infallible path to inner peace. It does not magically dissolve anger, anxiety, or fear. It puts you in touch with your inner self, and that is enough.

In order to maintain a relative efficiency, we learn to suppress whatever it may be that is troubling to us at the moment. But when you do Tai Chi it is impossible to avoid your own internal state. Practice for an hour and you will learn exactly how you feel, for better or worse. But if you can recognize and experience the pressure, or the unease, or whatever, at least you have a chance to live through it and to dissipate it.

A confusing but common experience is to emerge from a peaceful hour of practice, congratulating yourself on your "high", only to find yourself unbearably irritated by your next encounter with a surly bus driver. You call yourself a fake and write it off. But what has happened is the first step. Your defenses were down, and of course you were vulnerable. Tai Chi, like any spiritual discipline, offers us this first look within — a look at the garbage we have been collecting and storing away for years. There is no way around it, only, some day, through it. Day by day, the slow, soothing motion dissolves the physical tensions and obstructions. Physical ease reverberates through the soul.

The spiritual ideal of Tai Chi remains, for most of us, just that — an ideal. Do you know any real person with the total acceptance of the mythical Sage for whom "life is no better than death?" We wish to be wise and transcendentally detached, but who is truly immune from grief at the death of a lover or friend? An ideal is something to move towards. Tai Chi is a kind of counter-pull, which throws into relief the outlines of our confused desire, our ambitions, our angers. It takes us for a short time on a visit to another kind of inner world.

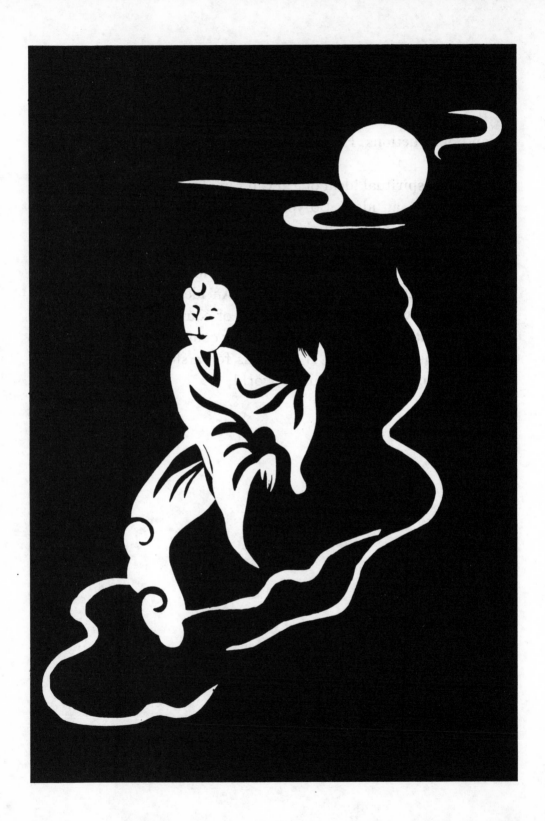

The Long Form

We are rooted in a place; we are rooted in the absence of a place. Between the two is the breathing of a shadow. There, for me, the Tai Chi Ch'uan unfolds.

"Shadow Boxing: Reflections on the Tai Chi Chuan".
Herbert Blau 1970

The experience of Tai Chi makes sense only in time, for it is the continuity of movement that gives life to the form. The quality of each instant is that of transition, of change — from one leg to the other, from up to down, forward to backward, inhaling to exhaling. There are no corners, no high points, no moments at which the movement is more fully realized than at others.

The continuity and clarity of the movements are bound up with the image of the circle, and in our movements while practicing the form we use our bodies to

39

describe and articulate these circular movements in space. In some ways it makes no more sense to show an instant of movement captured on film and to represent it as Tai Chi than to take a small portion of a circle and use it to represent the circle itself. It takes considerable imagination to recreate the whole from the part, and consequently we believe that it is misleading to pretend that Tai Chi can be taught in a book.

We have, however, included close to two hundred photographs which represent ten minutes of continuous movement. Our intention in presenting these photographs of the form which we practice is to make it available for purposes of comparison to students who know different forms, and to students of "The Long Form" who can use these photographs to refine their own movements.

"The Long Form", the first section of which is presented in these photographs, is performed by H. H. Lui.

"THE LONG FORM"
SEQUENCE OF MOVEMENTS IN THREE PARTS

N, E, S, W are North, East, South, and West.

PART I

1. Preparatory Period (N)
2. Commencement of Tai Chi Chuan (N)
3. Right (N E), Left (N W) Pull Down
4. Left Push Hand (W)

 5. Fan Through the Back (N W)
 6. Stab Hand (N W)
 7. Right Turn, Ward Off, Grasp Bird's Tail & Apparent Close UP (S E)
 8. Left Turn, Ward Off, Grasp Bird's Tail & Apparent Close UP (N E)
 9. Right Step Up & Pull Down (E)
10. Left Single Whip (W)
11. Right (N W), Left (S W) Pull Down, Elbow-stroke & Shoulder-stroke
12. Right Step Forward & Push Palm (W)
13. Step Back & Stork Cools Its Wings (W)
14. Left Brush Knee, Twist Step & Play the Fiddle (W)
15. Turn, Right Brush Knee, Twist Step & Play the Fiddle (N)
16. Turn, Left Brush Knee, Twist Step & Play the Fiddle (S)
17. Turn, Right Pull Down, Deflect Downward, Parry,
         Punch & Apparent Close Up (N W)
18. Turn, Left Pull Down, Deflect Downward, Parry,
         Punch & Apparent Close Up (S W)
19. Turn & Carry Tiger to Mountain (N)

PART II

 1. Right (E), Left (N E), Climb Mountain on Tiger Back
 2. Right Turn, Three Palm Movements, Grasp Bird's Tail
         & Apparent Close Up (S W)
 3. Left Turn, Three Palm Movements, Grasp Bird's Tail
         & Apparent Close Up (N E)
 4. Right Step Up & Pull Down (E)
 5. Left Semi-Single Whip (W)
 6. Left (S W), Right (N W), Push Mountain Into Sea
 7. Left (S), Right (N), Horizontal Elbow Movements
 8. Left, Right Fist Under Elbow (W)
 9. Left, Right, Repulse Monkey (W)
10. Left, Right, Step Forward, Brush Arm & Push Palm (W)
11. Right Push Hand (N)
12. Right Fan Through the Back (N W)
13. Elbow-stroke & Shoulder-stroke (N W)
14. Left Pull Down, Elbow-stroke & Shoulder-stroke (S E)
15. Right Step Forward & Push Palm (W)

16. Step Back & Left Stork Cools Its Wings (W)
17. Left Brush Knee & Twist Step (W)
18. Right Pull Up Curtain (W)
19. Right Needle at Sea Bottom (W)
20. Right Green Dragon Darts Out from Water (W)
21. Right Turn Around & Chop Fist (E)
22. Right Turn, Ward Off, Grasp Bird's Tail & Apparent Close Up (S E)
23. Left Turn, Ward Off, Grasp Bird's Tail & Apparent Close Up (N E)
24. Right Step Up & Pull Down (E)
25. Left Single Whip (W)
26. First Style Wave Hands Like Clouds (W)
27. Left Single Whip (W)
28. Step Up (W), Right High Pat on Horse (W), Left Snake Creeps
       Down (S W) & Separation of Right Foot (N W)
29. Step Back, Left High Pat on Horse (W), Right Snake Creeps
       Down (N W) & Separation of Left Foot (S W)
30. Left Turn & Kick Left Foot (E)
31. Left Brush Knee & Twist Step (E)
32. Step Forward, Right, Left Brush Knee & Groin Punch (E)
33. Turn, Creep Down & Right Turn Over Hands (W)
34. Step Up & Left Turn Over Hands (S)
35. Right Fist Under Elbow (S)
36. Kick Right Foot (S W)
37. Turn Around & Right Pat on Horse (N W)
38. Creep Down (S E), & Hit Tiger At Left (S)
39. Turn & Hit Tiger at Right (N)
40. Full Down & Kick Right Foot (N)
41. Right & Left, Double Fists (N)
42. Pull Down, Turn & Kick Left Foot (S)
43. Right Turn & Subdue Tiger (S)
44. Step Forward in Yin-Yang Steps (W)
45. Right Ward Off, Follow with Left Punch & Apparent Close Up (N W)
46. Left Ward Off, Follow with Right Punch & Apparent Close Up (S W)
47. Turn & Carry Tiger to Mountain (N)

PART III

1. Left (W), Right (N W), Climb Mountain on Tiger Back

2. Left Turn, Three Palm Movements, Grasp Bird's Tail & Apparent Close Up (S E)
3. Left Turn, Three Palm Movements, Grasp Bird's Tail & Apparent Close Up (N E)
4. Right Turn, Step Up & Pull Down (S W)
5. Left Slanting Single Whip (N E)
6. Left (N E) & Right (S E), Partition of Wild Horse Mane
7. Turn & Push Palm (E)
8. Left Turn, Ward Off, Grasp Bird's Tail & Apparent Close Up (W)
9. Turn & Horizontal Palm Movement (N)
10. Right Turn, Ward Off, Grasp Bird's Tail & Apparent Close Up (N E)
11. Left Turn, Step Up & Pull Down (S W)
12. Right Slanting Single Whip (N E)
13. Right (N E), Left (S W), Right (N W) & Left (S E) (Four Corners) Fair Lady Works at Shuttles
14. Right Step Back, Ward Off, Grasp Bird's Tail & Apparent Close Up (S E)
15. Left Turn, Ward Off, Grasp Bird's Tail & Apparent Close Up (N E)
16. Right Step Up & Pull Down (E)
17. Left Single Whip (W)
18. Second Style Wave Hands Like Clouds (W)
19. Left Single Whip & Creep Down (W)
20. Step Up & Golden Cock Stands on One (Left) Leg (W)
21. Step Back & Gold Cock Stands on One (Right) Leg (W)
22. Kick Left Foot, Left & Right, Repulse Monkey (W)
23. Right (N W) & Left (S W) Pull Down & Separation of Palms
24. Left Fan Through the Back (S W)
25. Left Elbow-stroke & Shoulder-stroke (S W)
26. Right Pull Down, Elbow-stroke & Shoulder-stroke (N W)
27. Left Step Forward & Push Palm (W)
28. Step Back & Right Stork Cools Its Wings (W)
29. Right Brush Knee & Twist Step (W)
30. Left Pull Up Curtain (W)
31. Left Needle at Sea Bottom (W)
32. Left Green Dragon Darts Out from Water (W)
33. Left Turn Around & Chop Fist (E)
34. Left Fist Under Elbow (S E)

35. Kick Left Foot (S E), Turn Around & Left Pat on Horse (N W)
36. Right Turn, Ward Off, Grasp Bird's Tail & Apparent Close Up (S E)
37. Left Turn, Ward Off, Grasp Bird's Tail & Apparent Close Up (N E)
38. Right Step Up & Pull Down (E)
39. Left Single Whip (W)
40. Third Style Wave Hands Like Clouds (W)
41. Left Single Whip (W)
42. Step Forward & Right High Pat on Horse (W)
43. Step Forward & Left White Snake Puts Out Its Tongue (W)
44. Step Back & Right Single Whip (W)
45. Step Forward & Left High Pat on Horse (W)
46. Step Forward & Right White Snake Puts Out Its Tongue (W)
47. Turn & Push Palm (N W)
48. Turn, Right Cross Legs & Punch Downward (S E)
49. Stand Up, Left Cross Legs & Punch Downward (N E)
50. Step Back, Right Dragon Stretches Its Claws, Cobra Turns Over Its Body & White Ape Offers Fruits (S E)
51. Step Back Left Dragon Stretches Its Claws, Cobra Turns Over Its Body & White Ape Offers Fruits (N E)
52. Right Dragon Stretches Its Claws (E) & Push Palm (E)
53. Left Turn, Ward Off, Grasp Bird's Tail & Apparent Close Up (W)
54. Step Forward, Right Ward Off, Grasp Bird's Tail & Apparent Close Up (N W)
55. Turn & Right Single Whip (W)
56. Snake Creeps Down, Stand Up & Left High Pat on Horse (W)
57. Step Up & Right Seven Star Fists (W)
58. Step Back & Left Stork Cools Its Wings (W)
59. Turn with a "Hundred Times Trained" Leg (W)
60. Step Back, Left & Right, Ride Tiger (W)
61. Left & Right, Shoot Tiger with Bow (N W)
62. Step Up, Creep Down, Step Forward, Right Ward Off, Follow with Left Punch & Apparent Close Up (N W)
63. Left Step Up, Creep Down, Step Forward, Left Ward Off, Follow with Right Punch & Apparent Close Up (S W)
64. Turn & Carry Tiger to Mountain (N)
65. Conclusion of Grand Terminus (Tai-Chi)

The Long Form

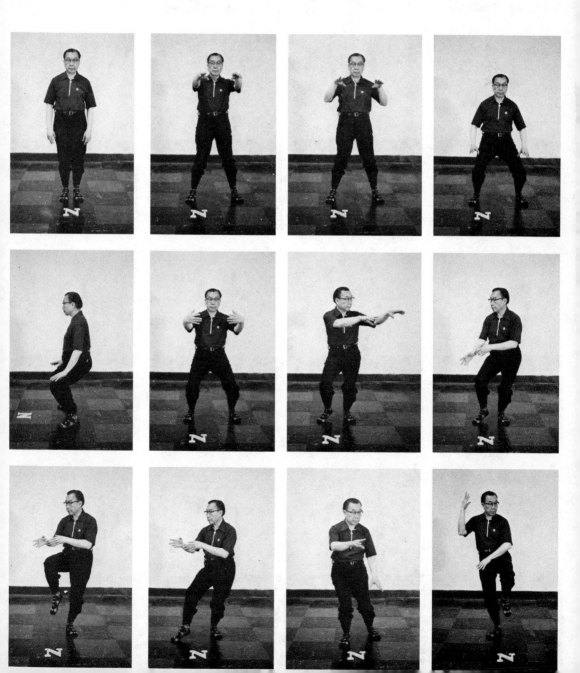

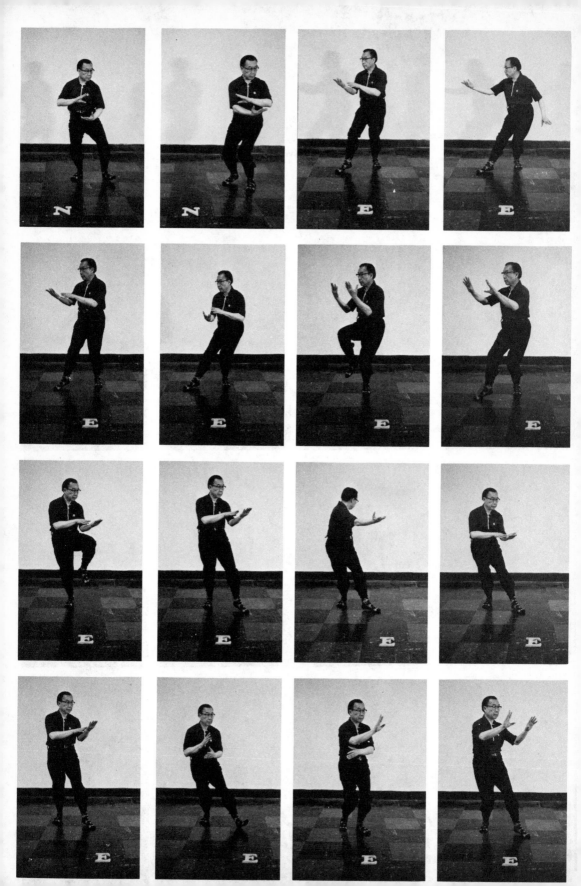

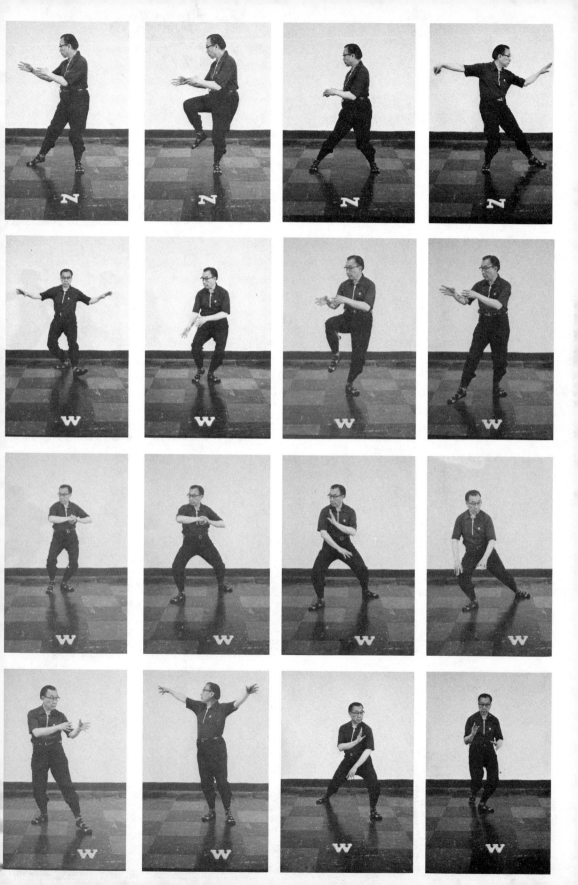

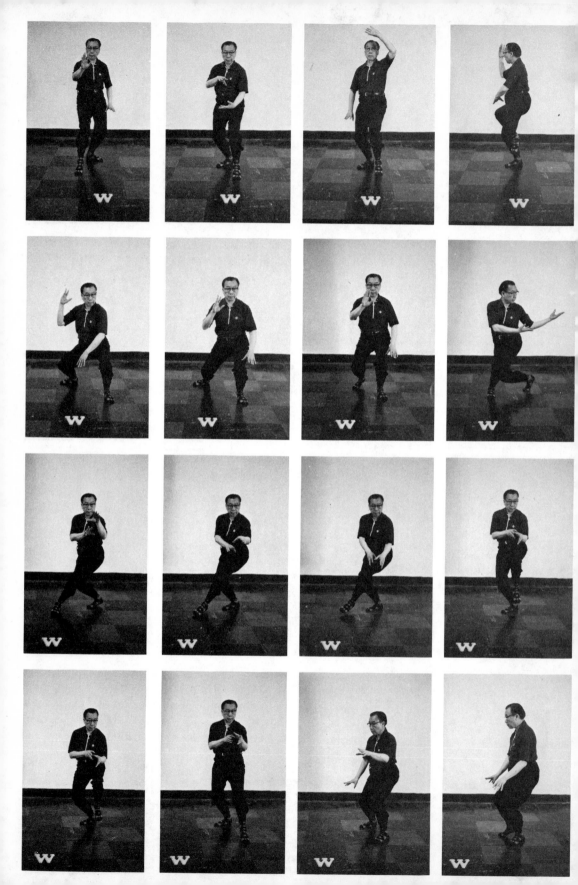

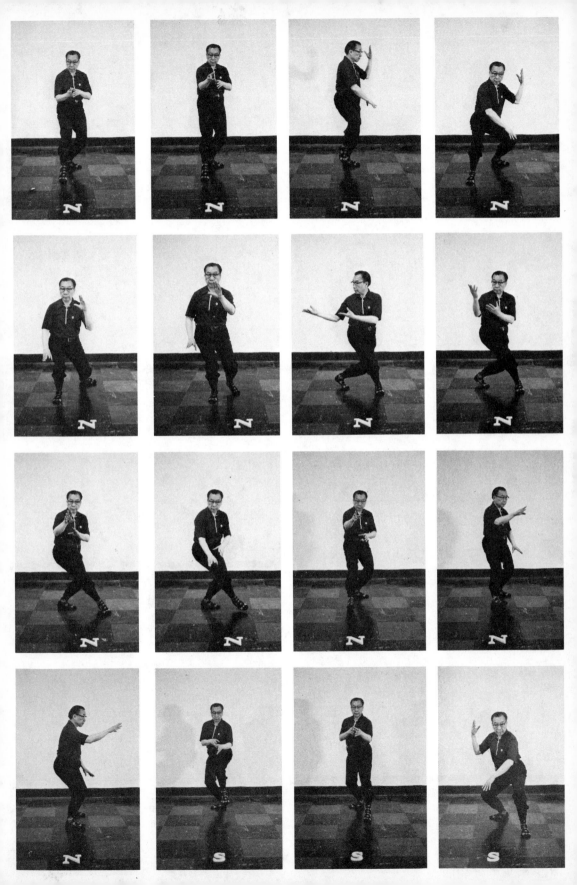

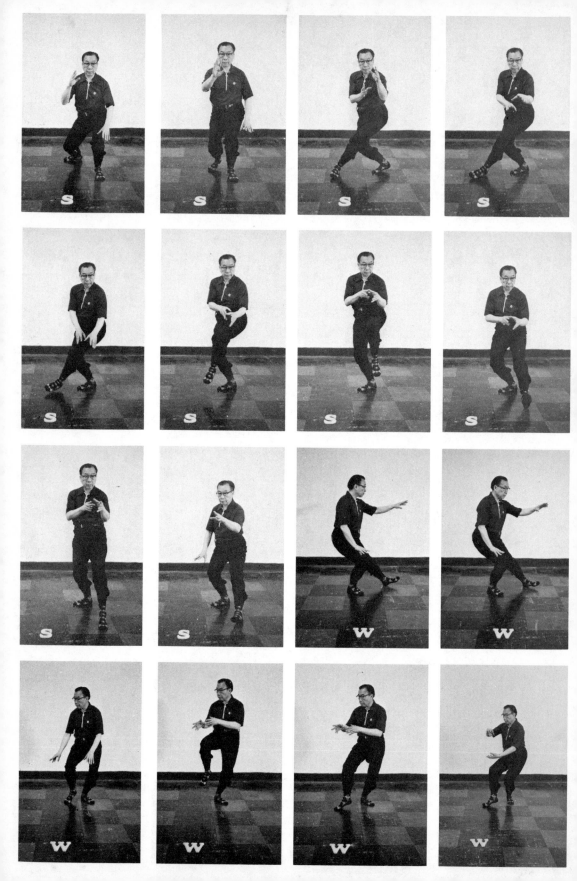

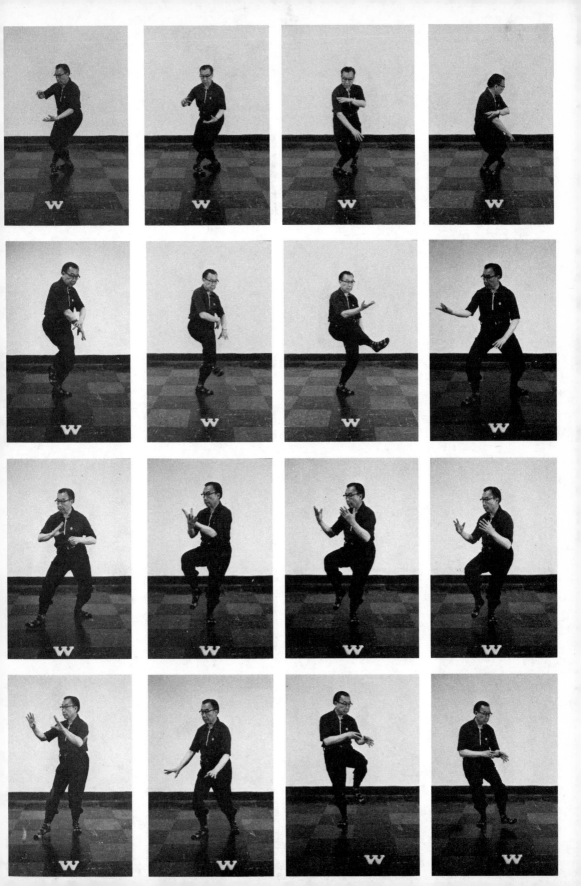

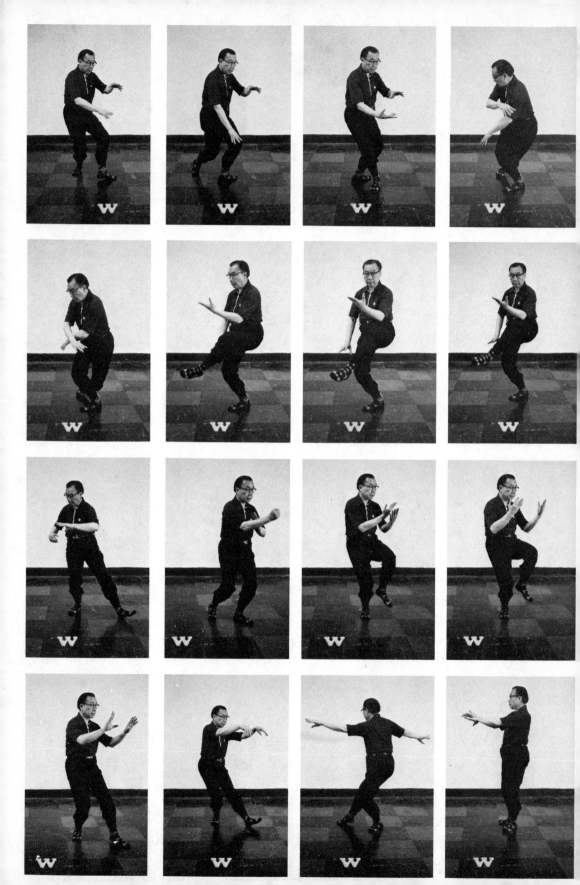

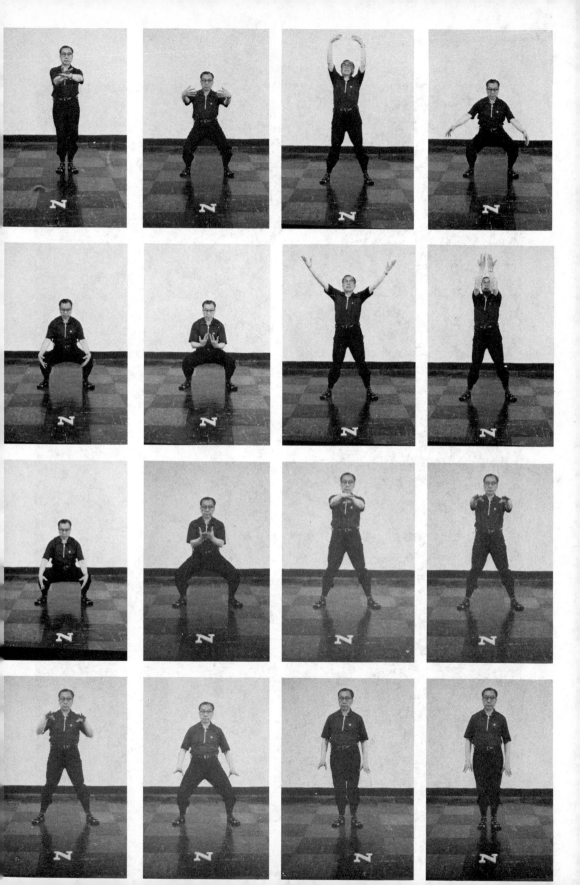

The History of Tai Chi Ch'uan and an Introduction to the "Classics"

The historical origins of Tai Chi are obscure at best; most of the available genealogies of Tai Chi masters are impossibly confusing to the English reader. This summary is intended to convey the flavor of the legends without getting involved in interminable arguments about the accuracy of dates and names. Some of the most appealing stories are probably the most apocryphal. The traditional lore is verbal, as well as written. We have included some of these stories, called in Chinese "wild history", in the belief that mythology is as informative as history and that it is not always necessary to be able to distinguish between them.

Chinese physical culture begins before history. A leg-

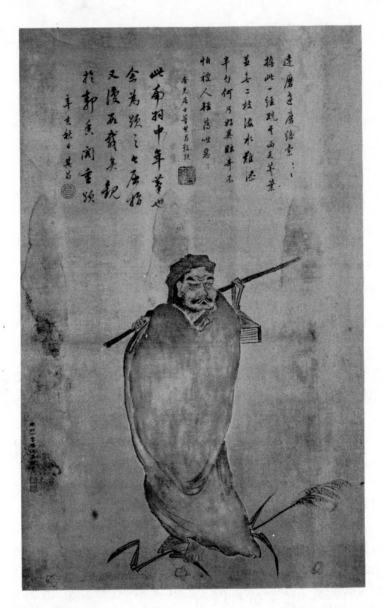

Bodhidharma. Original painting by Feng Tien. Ch'ing Dynasty.
Courtesy of Field Museum of Natural History, Chicago.

endary philosopher king of the forty-sixth century B.C., said to have created the original eight trigrams of the *I Ching*, ordered the performance of a Great Dance to help cure the people of disease. The ancient association of exercise with therapeutic and preventative medicine predates the development of the martial arts. The "Father of Chinese medicine" (190 A.D.) invented and taught a series of exercises based on the postures of animals. Many of the "steps" of Tai Chi also take their names from animals, real or mythical — "carry the tiger to the mountain", "repulse the monkey", "the dance of the dragon", etc.

The history of the martial arts in China begins with Bodhidharma (Ta-Mo), who came to China from India, teaching a kind of Buddhism that was a forerunner of what we know as Zen, or Ch'an Buddhism in China. He was concerned with the physical health of the monks, since they spent so many of their days in sedentary meditation. The exercise that he created was called Shao-Lin Ch'uan, after the Shao-Lin monastery. Other stories about the origins of the martial arts mention the need for a means of self-defense in disordered and violent times, since monks were not permitted to carry arms. For everyone, not only monks, the art of fighting was more of a genuine necessity before the widespread use of firearms reduced it to the status of a sport, albeit a deadly one.

The acknowledged "creator" of Tai Chi was a Taoist monk, Chang San-feng, who reworked the original forms of Shao-Lin with a new emphasis on breathing and in-

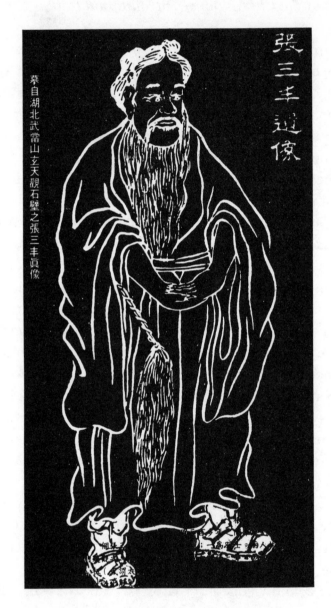

張三丰遺像

摹自湖北武當山玄天觀石壁之張三丰眞像

Chang Sang-feng, the reputed founder of Tai Chi Ch'uan, and a Taoist monk.

58

ner control. He lived sometime between the twelfth and fourteenth centuries A.D. His actual existence is unverifiable. He is the Paul Bunyan of Tai Chi, larger than life in every way. By some calculations he lived for over two hundred years. He could walk thousands of miles without getting tired, and without blinking an eye he could catch in one hand the arrows of his enemies. He had a pet ape who collected firewood and practiced a simian version of Tai Chi. The story has it that Tai Chi was revealed to Chang during a noon-time meditation. Looking out of the window, he saw a magpie trying to attack a snake. The snake teased the bird, managing always to be just out of reach, curling around and around in spirals, as snakes are wont to do. Thus the essence of Tai Chi — the inviolate nature of the circle. Chang Sang-feng marks the division of Chinese pugilism into two schools: soft and hard, or inner and outer, Nei Chia and Wai Chia. The earliest written work on Tai Chi is attributed to Chang. However, the authorship of the early "classics" will always be in doubt (not that it makes much difference), owing to the oriental tradition of deference to ancestral authority. Many writers were reluctant to affix their own names to their work, considering it less presumptuous to attribute it to some historically recognized expert.

In any case, the next name that appears is that of Wang Chung-yueh. Originally it was believed that he lived in the thirteenth century; later evidence places him in the eighteenth century. A school-teacher by profession, he and his pupil Chiang Fa were the teachers of the Ch'en family. Supposedly, Chang San-feng created the thirteen postures, said to correspond with the eight trigrams of the *I Ching* and the five basic elements of ancient Chinese cosmology. (There have been several books written in English which purport to explain the relationship of the cosmology to the exercise. The basic equivalence remains unclear to these Western readers. The correspondence of the movements to the elements, or to the trigrams, appears to be one of arbitrary coincidence.) Wang is credited with linking these original postures together to make a continuous sequence of movement. Two of the classical theoretical works are attributed to Wang. They are said to have been discovered in a small salt shop in Wu Yang in the nineteenth century.

One of the difficulties in tracing the history of Tai Chi is that the tradition is a curious blend of popular lore, largely unrecorded, and the secret, carefully-guarded heritage of the elite, upper-class families. After Wang Chung-yueh (or before, depending on which dates you accept), one form of the exercise was kept inside the family of Ch'en for fourteen generations. The privileged family grew lazy and indolent, to the despair of their teacher. An enterprising servant taught himself Tai Chi by watching through a crack in the wall. When the servant successfully demonstrated his competence, the astonished teacher accepted him as a disciple. Horatio Alger, Chinese Style. (This story also occurs in reverse form. A

teacher in Peking at the beginning of the Nationalist re-
gime claimed that he was a descendent of the Tsung family of the Tang dynasty and had learned a secret family
form. It is suspected that he created his own exercise and
fabricated the family tree in order to give his teachings
the necessary voice of authority.)

Yang Lu-chan, the ambitious servant, eventually became a famous teacher in Peking. There he taught Tai
Chi publicly for the first time, in the latter half of the
nineteenth century. Called Yang The Unsurpassed, he had
two sons whom he brow-beat mercilessly in the name of
his art. Despite, or perhaps because of, the paternal
pressure, the sons showed little aptitude for the exercise
during their father's lifetime. After his death one of
Yang's students, not a member of the family, proclaimed
at the graveside that he was the legitimate heir to the
legacy of Tai Chi. The real sons were roused from their
apathy by jealous fury and devoted themselves hence-
forward to diligent study and practice. In later years the
three were happily reconciled and continued teaching
in peace.

Tai Chi is customarily divided into different styles
or forms, identified by family names. (In Chinese the
family name comes first.) The style called Yang, after
Yang Lu-chan, is the most widespread today. The Yang
style is firmer and more expansive that the Wu style, the
second most popular. However, the forms are not en-
tirely distinguishable one from another, since the various

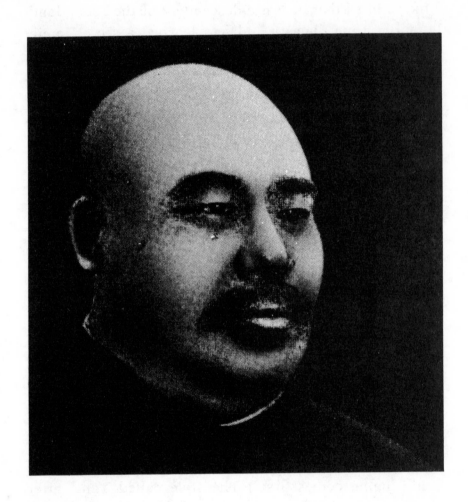

Yang Ching-pu (1883–1936) was the grandson of the founder of the Yang School. He is credited with stabilizing the Yang style when he became chief instructor of the family.

62

strains of teachings are crisscrossed and interconnected. "The Long Form", illustrated in this book, combines qualities of Yang and the smaller, more subtle Wu style. Within the generic divisions of Yang and Wu there are countless different sequences being taught today, since most masters adapt their own forms, either condensing or elaborating, through the course of long years of teaching.

The teaching has traditionally been conservative, passed on from father to son, with very few notable exceptions. The student demonstrates his devotion by his unquestioning obedience; there are no explanations and signs of "frivolity" are not tolerated. This has created a long history of teacher/student schisms. Since there is no room for questioning, creative students often have been forced to break with their teachers.

However, the specific movements and the order of the sequence is not the most important thing. In the earliest writing on the theory of Tai Chi, Chang says, "Ultimately, everything depends on one's will or mind and not on the external appearance of the movements." The significant thing is the internal experience — any form is legitimate if it adheres to the basic principles contained in a small number of documents known as "The Tai Chi Classics." We have included some of these here, translated by H. H. Lui. For readers who are unfamiliar with Tai Chi, a casual reading of the Classics will give a general introduction to the exercise. For serious students it is necessary to return again and again to the Classics in order to keep in touch with the images that give life and meaning to the movement.

The classics are not entertaining bed-time reading — they are brief, reflective notes that will change with each reading, like Tai Chi itself. They combine precise technical instruction with vivid imagery. Read in a spirit of emptiness and ease they will resonate and echo through your daily living. They are deceptive in their simplicity. At first glance, all is obvious. But with attention and re-reading the puzzles begin to unfold and reveal themselves.

The special beauty of Tai Chi is its integration of the physical with the . . . call it mental, spiritual, psychological, whatever. If the student has no understanding of the principles, it is just an empty form, in the most negative sense of that word, and long years of practice will be in vain. It is the image that brings together mind and body. "If beginners can comprehend the truth in . . . theory they will not easily get tired of it although the path to learning it appears simple and tasteless." The crucial concept is "ideation" — the mind leads the body by imagining, or contemplating, each move in the split second before it happens. The intention exists before the gesture, and continues after it, linking it to the next one.

Many people practice Tai Chi solely for health and meditation, and yet the Classics refer often to the "opponent". The technique of self-defense overlaps here with the philosophy of exercise — what is most effective in a fight is also most conducive to good health, long life, and mental serenity. This is not just a curious coincidence. It implies a coherent vision of life that includes self-protection. The world is viewed as an ever-changing interplay of forces. Each creature seeks to realize its own nature; to find its place in the universe. Not to conquer, but to endure. The assumption is that there *are* hostile forces. One can be attacked by animals, by angry or arrogant people, or just by the forces of Nature, within and without. In the human world attack is verbal and emotional as often as it is physical. The most subtle and manipulative struggles are the ones of which we are least conscious. But the prescription for survival is always the same — integrity. This is more than a moral adage, it is a physical actuality.

The central image is water. It flows, filling in available space, rounding out hollows; it closes over, liquid but impenetrable. Beneath the surface is immeasureable depth. Water is a medium for power. Propelled with energy, water is as strong a force as dynamite. It yields, and yet recoils. The softness of Tai Chi is not spiritless or lethargic — it is the supple and resilient integrity of water.

The "form" of Tai Chi is not a fixed method; it is only a means. The body trains itself to become free, to learn keenness of sensation and a visceral understanding of force. The lesson of Tai Chi is primarily a strategic one. Force is neutralized through tranquility and the willingness to yield. This tactical advice is difficult for the Western ear to hear. It is truly a foreign procedure, for most of us. The self — sacrificed, emptied, neutral — devotes itself to understanding and following the opponent. Strength and speed, the conventional fighting virtues, are replaced by sensitivity. The opponent attacks, you retreat; the opponent retreats; you follow, sticking like glue. In the practice of the solo exercise, the opponent becomes imaginary, a symbol of a physical and mental reality. The space around the body is like water, and the currents gently push and pull. Boxing with its shadow, the body generates its own rhythm of advance and retreat.

In reading the Classics (and learning Tai Chi), it is not enough to accept and agree. It is necessary to understand the very real difference between the way of Tai Chi and our own style of being. Modern popular psychology is a potent, insidious force. It colors our shared consciousness, whether or not we accept it on a rational level. Confrontation is the most popular current mode of human interaction. Self-expression is all; "repression" is the villain. "Let it all hang out", etc. Tai Chi has been used in the service of these clichés, but its method is actually much more subtle, more elusive. The "inner energy" of Tai Chi is not visible. True vitality is conceived of as being beneath the surface. The strategic counsel of Tai Chi is to yield rather than to resist. Of course we have all had moments when honest, outright resistance was the only possible response. But the advice is procedural, tactical. It helps us to recognize which moment requires which response.

For an American there are many obstacles in the way of a living understanding of Tai Chi. Most of us are susceptible to the need for success and the demands of speed and efficiency in order to compete successfully. And there are many aspects of our own cultural style which we may not care to discard, no matter how green the grass may look on the other side of the Great Wall. This question — what can Tai Chi mean for us — is central to our book and the subject of many of the later essays. But first the reader must meet the Classics, undistracted by our interpretations.

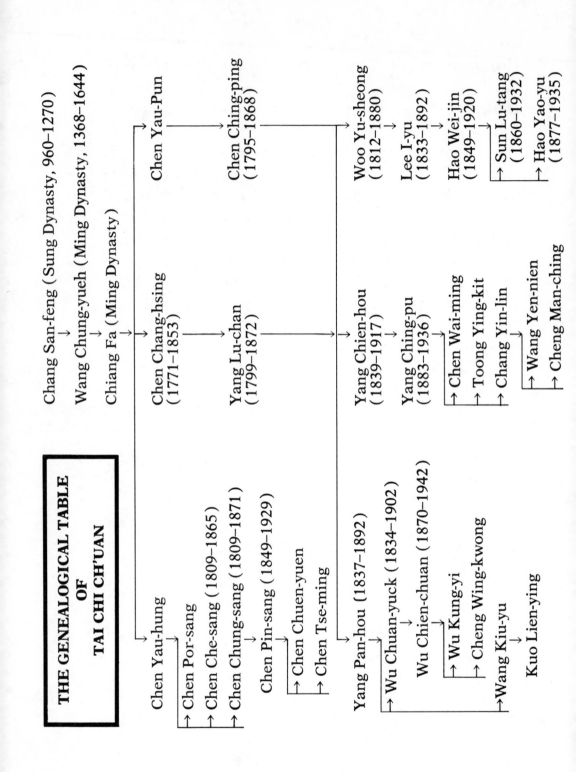

THE GENEALOGICAL TABLE OF TAI CHI CH'UAN

Chang San-feng (Sung Dynasty, 960–1270)
↓
Wang Chung-yueh (Ming Dynasty, 1368–1644)
↓
Chiang Fa (Ming Dynasty)
↓

Chen Yau-Pun → Chen Ching-ping (1795–1868) → Woo Yu-sheong (1812–1880)
→ Lee I-yu (1833–1892)
→ Hao Wei-jin (1849–1920)
→ Sun Lu-tang (1860–1932)
→ Hao Yao-yu (1877–1935)

Chen Chang-hsing (1771–1853) → Yang Lu-chan (1799–1872) → Yang Chien-hou (1839–1917)
→ Yang Ching-pu (1883–1936)
→ Chen Wai-ming
→ Toong Ying-kit
→ Chang Yin-lin
→ Wang Yen-nien
→ Cheng Man-ching

Chen Yau-hung
→ Chen Por-sang
→ Chen Che-sang (1809–1865)
→ Chen Chung-sang (1809–1871)

Chen Pin-sang (1849–1929)
→ Chen Chuen-yuen
→ Chen Tse-ming

Yang Pan-hou (1837–1892)
→ Wu Chuan-yuck (1834–1902)
→ Wu Chien-chuan (1870–1942)
→ Wu Kung-yi
→ Cheng Wing-kwong

→ Wang Kiu-yu
→ Kuo Lien-ying

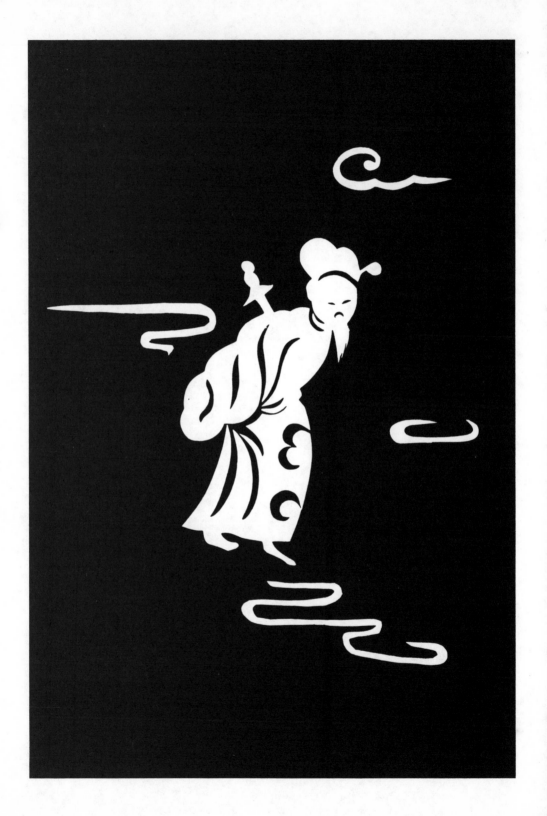

Tai Chi Ch'uan Classics

TRANSLATOR'S NOTE

Nature is always in motion. Man also should strengthen himself without interruption.

I Ching

Are you able to gather your intrinsic energy to attain the suppleness of a new-born baby?

Lao Tzu

Mencius said, "The power and vision of Le Low and the skill of King-shoo, without the compass and square could not form squares and circles." Without the classical writings of the originator Chang San-feng and his remarkable follower, Wang Chung-yueh, Tai Chi Ch'uan would virtually lack its "compass and square". Therefore, when

71

students of mine asked me for an acceptable yardstick for measuring the accuracy of the exercise, I referred them to the study of the three most important treatises on Tai Chi Ch'uan, attributed to Chang and Wang, as well as the ten essential points of Yang Ching-pu, the leader of the famous Yang School, and the six essential points of Wu Chien-chuan, leader of the renowned Wu School. For prudent students of Tai Chi Ch'uan these classical works are something they must not only taste or chew but digest.

In the summer of 1971 when I vacationed in San Francisco I visited on many occasions the old master of Tai Chi Ch'uan, Kuok Lien-ying. Each time we met he stressed the importance of the Tai Chi Ch'uan Classics. In his book *Tai Chi Ch'uan Theory and Practice*, in Chinese, Kuok quoted his master, Wang Kiu-yu, as follows:

> In the practice of Tai Chi Ch'uan it matters little from what school or what master one learns; the number of movements in a version, a few movements more or a few movements less; and the type of form or circle, high form or low form, big circle or small circle. These are all up to the individual. As long as one does not deviate from the basic principles set forth in The Classics, one can reap the same benefits from the exercise and become a successful performer.

Another old master, Cheng Man-ching of New York, held a view similar to Kuok's. In his book *Tai-Chi* Cheng observed.

72

The Classics are our best link with the past of Tai Chi. They are the basis of the art. By their nature they are discursive and redundant, but, at the same time, profound. In the present era, when Tai Chi has proliferated into so many schools, The Classics can be used as a model. If these systems violate The Classics, the systems are wrong.

For these reasons, it is my sincere hope that this translation will give students a better understanding of the philosophy behind the exercise and thus enable them to enjoy good health and longevity.

While continuity in movement is a fundamental characteristic of Tai Chi Ch'uan, constancy in practice every day, month after month and year after year, is the road to one's success in the exercise. It is indeed a long journey. However, in the words of Lao Tzu: "A journey of a thousand miles starts from where your feet stand." Let us begin today.

H. H. Lui

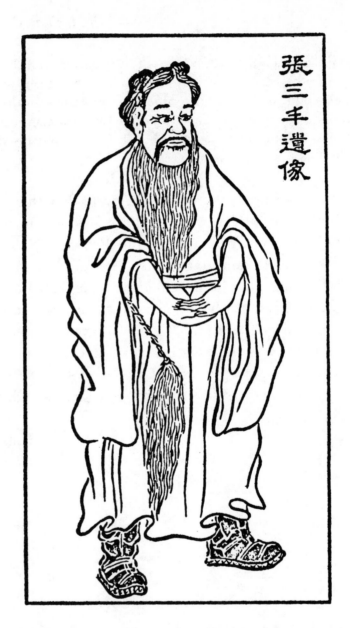

張三丰遺像

Chang San-feng, the Taoist priest of Wu Tang Mountain. Credited with being the founder of Tai Chi Ch'uan in the thirteenth century.

74

CHANG SAN-FENG'S TREATISE ON TAI CHI CH'UAN

> *The original text of Yang Lu-chan — one of the great nineteenth century masters — says that this treatise was the work of the originator of Tai Chi Ch'uan, Chang San-feng, a Taoist priest of Wu Tang Mountain in the thirteenth century. It was Chang San-feng's hope that heroes all over the world would enjoy good health and longevity by practicing Tai Chi, and that the art be practiced as more than just a martial skill.*

In each movement the whole body must be light and nimble. More important still, all movements must be continuous.

The intrinsic energy or "chi" should circulate actively. The spirit should be retained internally.

Let no part of the movement indicate imperfection — neither over-expanding or caving in — nor should there be any discontinuity.

In all movements the inner strength is rooted in the feet, developed in the thighs, controlled by the waist, and expressed through the fingers. From the feet *to* the thigh, *to* the waist, and *to* the fingers there must be complete coordination so that whether you are in advance or in retreat you will be in a favorable position. If you find yourself in an unfavorable position, your body will appear scattered and confused, and the fault can be traced to the waist and thighs. In all movements, such as upwards, downwards, forwards, and backwards, the same significance of the waist and thighs holds true.

However, ultimately everything depends on one's will or mind, and not on the external appearance of the movements.

In any movement when there is up, there must be down; when there is front, there must be rear; and when there is left, there must be right. If one wishes to execute an upward movement, it must be preceded by a downward one. This like the idea of uprooting an object — the first thing you do is to push it down. Since the root of the object is lifted, it follows that it is ready to be toppled.

The two complementary factors, emptiness and solidness, must be distinctly differentiated. In each and every inch of movement, these two factors are involved.

Every joint of the entire body must be strung together so that the body acts as an integrated unit without the least interruption. Each movement proceeds inch by inch without gaps or breaks in the continuity.

A TREATISE ON TAI CHI CH'UAN
BY WANG CHUNG-YUEH

> *It was believed that Wang Chung-yueh lived in the thirteenth century. There is some thought now that he actually lived in the middle of the eighteenth century. Wang is credited with combining the original thirteen postures into something resembling the present continuous forms of Tai Chi. Wu Yu-seong (1812-80) was given this manual by his brother, who discovered it in a salt shop. Based on the teachings in this manual Wu went on to teach and to form the Wu School. Wu made this treatise available to his students.*

Tai Chi has evolved from Wu Chi (The Void Terminus). It is the source of activity and inactivity and mother of the Yang and Yin.

[According to early Chinese cosmology, in the beginning was the great void, empty and without boundary. Then came the principles of Yang, or activity, and Yin, or inactivity. These in combination formed the Tai Chi.]

In movement the Yin and Yang act independently. In quietude, the two fuse into one. There should be no exceeding or falling short. You stick to your opponent's curve or withdrawal with an extension while yielding to his extension with a bending.

Tai Chi Ch'uan

When an opponent's hard force is met with a soft retreat, it is termed "evasion". To stick to a retreating opponent's motion is known as "adherence" or adhesion.

Answer fast action with fast action, and slow movement with slow movement. Although there are a myriad of variations, the basic principle remains the same.

From the stage of familiarity with the techniques comes the stage of a gradual understanding of the inner strength, and from the stage of understanding of the inner strength comes the state of spiritual illumination. However, without going through prolonged and serious practice, it is impossible to reach ultimate enlightenment.

Keep your neck erect and direct the crown of your head upward as if your head were suspended from above. Keep your spirits raised and you will lose all clumsiness and obtuseness in your movements. Allow your intrinsic energy to sink to the "tan-tien" which is a spot about three inches below the navel.

[The "tan-tien" corresponds to the Yogic chakra located at this point, and in numerous other traditions it is thought to be a center of power or energy.]

Avoid leaning or inclining your body in any direction. Manifest or conceal your movement so completely that your opponent finds it impossible to detect your intention. ["Know your enemy as well as yourself and you will be invincible" wrote the famous Chinese military strategist Sun Tze.]

Answer a solid intrusion on the left by emptying the left. Likewise, answer an aggressive force on the right by yielding the right. The more your opponent pushes upward or downward against you, the more he feels there is no limit to the emptiness he encounters. The more he advances against you, the more he feels the distance incredibly long. The more he retreats from you, the more he feels the dead end desperately close.

Your body should be so light and nimble that a feather could not land on it without being felt, and a fly could not alight on it without setting it in motion.

Your opponent is not able to detect your moves, but you are able to anticipate his. A hero finds himself without match because he is a master of these principles.

In the field of pugilism there are many schools. Irrespective of the differences among these schools, they all share a belief that the strong overcomes the weak and the fast overtakes the slow. However, this situation is due to natural abilities that require no study. Tai Chi is different.

A careful analysis of the case in which "A trigger force of a mere four taels manages to move an object weighing one thousand catties" reveals the truth that it is not always sheer strength that wins. When "an old man was able to defeat a group of youthful attackers" it was demonstrated that speed or numbers alone did not assure victory.

Stand as a poised scale and move like a wheel.

Avoid leaning your body to one side or there is a tendency to fall to that side. Avoid distributing your body weight on both feet or you can easily become a victim of "double weightedness", and your movements will be impeded.

Often it has been the case that, even after years of practice, one can still be easily subdued by an opponent. This is because one has not been made to fully realize the fault implied in "double weightedness". To remedy this defect, one must seek to know the principles of Yin and Yang. Under the Yin-Yang theory to adhere is to evade and to evade is to adhere, just as the Yin cannot separate from its complementary part the Yang, and the Yang cannot separate from its complementary part the Yin. It is only in the state in which the Yin and the Yang complement each other harmoniously that there is an understanding of the "inner strength".

After one understands *inner strength,* more practice will bring more proficiency. If one furthers one's study by silent meditation and thorough analysis, a level will be attained where one can execute all of the movements using only the will.

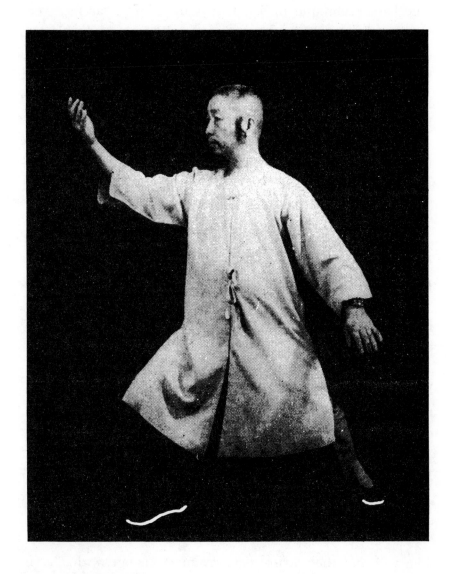

Cheng Man-ch'ing, one of the noted twentieth century masters, in the "Diagonal Flying Posture".

Tai Chi Ch'uan

The basic technique in Tai Chi is to learn to sacrifice your-self in order to follow your opponent. That is, not to initiate action against your opponent but to allow yourself to respond to whatever action your opponent takes. However, students often neglect this truth. How true is the old saying: "Devia-tion at the beginning of just a hair-breadth leads to a divergence of a thousand miles at the end". In the study of this art, there-fore, students should be sincere, thoughtful, and yielding.

AN EXPLANATION OF THE THIRTEEN POSTURES
BY WANG CHUNG-YUEH

Move your intrinsic energy with your mind so that it may sink and be gathered into your bones.

Permeate your body with your intrinsic energy in such a way that it may flow smoothly and be able to follow the direction of your mind.

If one's spirit can be lifted, there will be no sluggishness in movement. This is the meaning of "holding up the head straight as if it is suspended from above".

The will and the intrinsic energy must change with alacrity to insure roundness and swiftness in movement. This is termed 'the interplay of emptiness and solidness'.

82

To deliver strength one must remain calm and relaxed and allow the center of gravity to sink downward. One must be able to focus this energy in a single direction.

To be able to handle oncoming blows from all sides one must be still, remain centrally poised, well balanced, and expanded.

To circulate the intrinsic energy through the body one must act as if one were passing a thread through a pearl having nine zigzag paths: a slow and even course that leaves no corner untouched.

To develop strength one must act as if one were refining steel a hundred times so that nothing would be too hard for it to penetrate.

Poise your body like a hawk ready to pounce on a rabbit.
Alert your spirit like a cat ready to overtake a mouse.
In quietude be as still as a mountain.
In movement go like the current of a river.
Store strength as if releasing an arrow.
Seek straightness from the curve.
Store strength before releasing it.
Strength is delivered from the back.
Steps are changed in accordance with the change of postures.

To contract is to expand. Movement must be in absolute continuity. Back and forth must have folds and variations, advance and retreat must have turns and changes.

Tai Chi Ch'uan

Only when one can be extremely pliable and soft can one be extremely firm and hard.

Only when one truly knows how to inhale and exhale can one move nimbly and smoothly.

Intrinsic energy must be continuouly nourished. It can cause no harm.

Inner strength must be conserved in a curved way; then there will be excess to spare.

The mind is the commander; the intrinsic energy the flag; and the waist the banner.

One should first seek to stretch and expand and then seek to tighten and collect, and eventually one will reach a stage in which movements are so perfectly knitted together that one's defenses appear impenetrable.

It is said that if your opponent does not move, you do not move. If he makes the slightest move, you move ahead of him.

The inner strength may seem slack, but it is not. It may seem stretched but it is not. At times it may seem to have ceased, but at no time does it stop, for at all moments the will is active.

It is also said that the mind comes first and the body later. Keep

84

your stomach relaxed and soft and let the intrinsic energy permeate into your bones. Keep your spirit calm and easy and your body quiet. Under no circumstances let these facts slip from your mind.

Bear in mind that when one part of the body moves, all other parts of the body move. When one part of the body comes to a stand-still all other parts of the body come to a stand-still.

In all movements back and forth one must allow the intrinsic energy to adhere to the back and be gathered into the spine.

Internally one must strengthen the spirit. Externally one must exhibit one's genuine calmness.

Walk like a cat. Handle your inner strength as if you were reeling silk threads from a cocoon.

The aim of the whole body is to conserve spirit and not intrinsic energy. If one aims at conserving intrinsic energy the movements will be impeded. Whenever intrinsic energy becomes stagnant there can be no creation of true strength, only sheer hardness. Intrinsic energy is the rim of a wheel; the waist is the hub of the wheel.

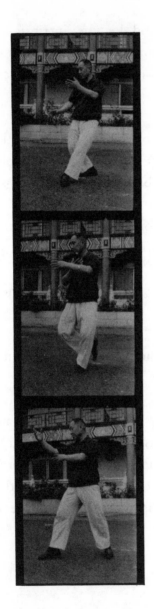
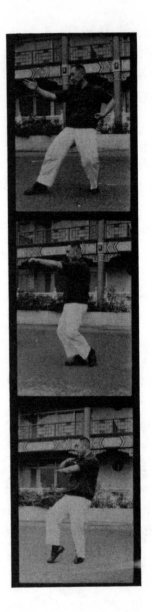

Wong Yen-nien, a contemporary Tai Chi Ch'uan master. Yang School.

86

THE TEN ESSENTIAL POINTS OF YANG CHING-PU

> *Yang Ching-pu (1883–1936) is credited with finally sta-*
> *bilizing the Yang style when he became the chief in-*
> *structor of the Yang Form. Yang Ching-pu was the*
> *grandson of the founder of the Yang School, Yang*
> *Lu-ch'an.*

I. *Suspend Your Head from Above and Keep It Up Straight*

By so doing your inner strength will be able to reach the crown
of your head and your spirit will be able to soar. But do not exert any force to attain this goal, for once you consciously or unconsciously apply force your neck will become stiff. A stiff neck,
regardless of the degree of stiffness, is an obstacle to the free
flowing of intrinsic energy and the smooth circulation of your
blood.

II. *Depress Your Chest and Raise Your Upper Back*

This posture will allow the intrinsic energy to sink into your
"tan-tien". Avoid pushing out your chest, for a "chest-out" position will cause your upper body to be heavy and your lower
body to be light. Also, your feet will then be subject to floating and you will have a hard time maintaining your body balance. By raising your upper back you attach your intrinsic
energy to your back enabling you to deliver your inner strength
effectively from your vertebrae.

Tai Chi Ch'uan

III. *Loosen Your Waist*

The waist is the key part of the body. Only when you are able to loosen your waist can you manage to keep your feet strong and your body secure and firm. Moreover, the change of steps from solid to empty or from empty to solid is all controlled by your waist. To execute this satisfactorily you must have a loosened waist. It was said, "The order for movement is issued from the waist", and "when your body appears scattered and lacks strength the remedy should be sought in your waist and legs".

IV. *Distinguish Between Solidness and Emptiness*

In the art of Tai Chi Ch'uan the differentiation between solidness and emptiness is of primary importance. When you rest your whole body weight on the right leg, your right leg is regarded as solid and your left leg as empty. On the other hand, when you rest your whole body weight on the left leg your left leg is regarded as solid and your right leg as empty. Only when you are able to distinguish solidness and emptiness can your movement be light and nimble. By no means need you exert. However, should you fail to make such distinctions your steps will be heavy and sluggish, and you can easily lose your body balance. Eventually you will become the victim of your opponent.

V. *Droop Your Shoulders and Sink Your Elbows*

By loosening your shoulder joints you allow your shoulders to droop downward. If your shoulders are raised they will block the intrinsic energy. Without the free flowing of intrinsic energy your movements will show a deficiency of inner strength and lack of continuity.

VI. *Apply Your Will and Not Your Force*

The Tai Chi Ch'uan Treatise said: "This is completely the use of your will and not your force". Therefore, while practicing you should totally relax your body and not permit the existence of any awkward force in your body to hinder your movement so that your movement can be light and nimble and you can act exactly as your mind directs. Someone may ask, "If one disregards the application of force, how can one develop strength?" It is because the system of veins and arteries in a human body is like the system of channels and streams on earth. Water runs smoothly when the channels and streams are not blocked; intrinsic energy flows freely when the veins and arteries are free from obstacles. If the body is filled with force the result is stagnation of the intrinsic energy and sluggishness in movement. When a part of the body gets stuck, the entire body suffers.

If one follows the rule to practice day after day for a long period of time, one will find that the use of will rather than force

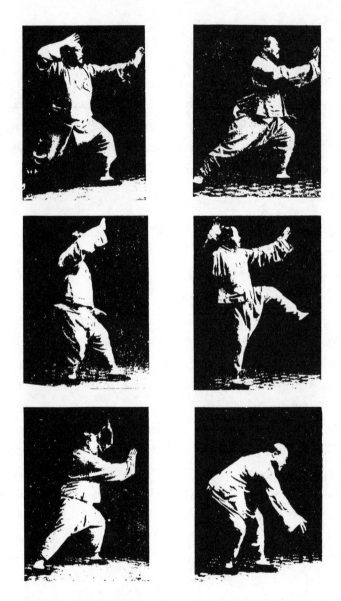

Yang Ching-pu (1883–1936). Leader of the Yang School, and a major figure in the history of modern Tai Chi Ch'uan.

90

results in the cultivation of inner strength. The Tai Chi Ch'uan treatise observed, "Extreme softness is conducive to extreme hardness". It is no surprise to find a Tai Chi expert with arms that are very soft in appearance but extremely hard inside — like two iron rods well wrapped with cotton. Thus, he can endure and withstand hardship in life.

VII. *Coordinate Your Upper and Lower Body Movements*

The Tai Chi Ch'uan Treatise said: "In all movement the inner strength is rooted in the feet, developed in the thighs, controlled by the waist, and expressed through the fingers. From the feet to the thighs, waist, and fingers there must be complete coordination and the whole body should act as one integrated unit". Therefore, when the hands move, the waist and the feet as well as the focus of the eyes, must move accordingly. This is the meaning of the coordination of the upper and lower body movements. Whenever there is a disagreement among any parts of the body the movement instantly will appear scattered and will lack strength.

VIII. *Unify Your Internal and External Movements*

Tai Chi trains the spirit of the individual. It was said, "The spirit is the master and the body is its servant". Therefore, when one manages to lift one's spirit one's movement will be light

91

and nimble. The nature of all movements consists of softness as well as hardness, and expansion as well as contraction. By expansion it does not mean expanding only the hands and the feet, but also the mind and the will. The same is true for contraction. Only when you can unify your internal and external movements can your body move as one integrated unit without interruption.

IX. *There Must Be Absolute Continuity in Your Movements*

In "Wai Chia" (Outer Intrinsic School) pugilism, the strength that is developed is a kind of awkward strength. ["Wai Chia" pugilism refers to the harder, more aggressive martial arts.] With this kind of strength there is a beginning and there is an end; there is discontinuity and there is interruption. It is not unusual under this system that when the old strength has been used up, new strength has not been developed. It is this "strength-gap" that gives one's opponent the advantage.

In Tai Chi (the "Nei Chia" or Inner Intrinsic School) *will* rather than *force* is applied to direct the body movements. From beginning to end the movements are continuous, without interruption. The end of one movement is the beginning of the next movement. In fact, there is no beginning or end within the circular movements of Tai Chi. It was said that Tai Chi Ch'uan acts in the manner of The Long River, the Yang Tze, which flows ceaselessly. It was also said that the action of the inner strength resembles the reeling of silk from a cocoon. All of these refer to the continuous nature of Tai Chi movements.

X. *Seek Serenity in Activity*

In "Wai Chia" pugilism the delivery of strength appears merely as a sort of "showing off". The practitioner demonstrates his ability and skill by exerting all his energy to jump or to firmly hold his position. Consequently, after practice, he usually feels very exhausted and tends to breathe rapidly. Tai Chi Ch'uan, on the other hand, aims at seeking serenity in activity. Though the practitioner is active externally, he is calm internally. In Tai Chi, the slower one executes the movements the better. For slowness in movement is conducive to deep and long breathing, and it enables the intrinsic energy to sink into the "tan-tien". In this situation the practitioner will not suffer from rapid breathing or troubles involving the heart or the circulation of blood.

If students of Tai Chi Ch'uan can carefully ponder these essential points they will be able to comprehend the true meaning of this exercise.

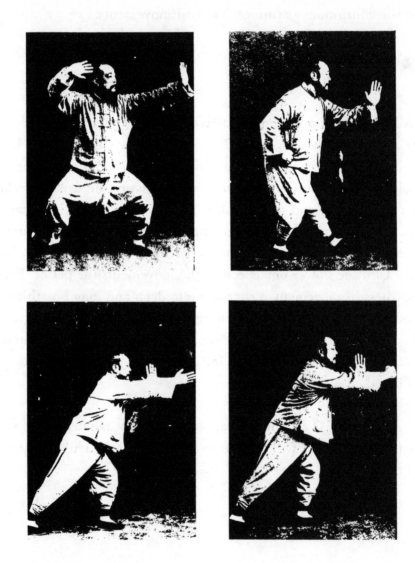

Master Wu Kam-Chuan.

94

THE SIX ESSENTIAL POINTS OF WU CHIEN-CHUAN

Wu Chien-chuan (1870–1942) was the leader of the well known Wu School of Tai Chi. The history of this style goes back to Chuan-yuck (1834–1902) who had studied with one of Yang Lu-ch'an's sons.

Tai Chi is unique in its cultivation of the practitioner's body and mind at the same time. Therefore, emphasis should be placed on the physical as well as the mental aspect while practicing the exercise.

The Physical Aspect

I. *The Suspension of the Head and the Lifting of the Inner Strength*

In practicing Tai Chi Ch'uan one must keep one's head in a central and erect position so that there is inner strength ascending to the crown of the head. The head is the key part of the entire body. Only when it is maintained in a central and erect position can one's spirit be raised and kept active. However, one must not apply force to attain this position. In order to do this effortlessly it is best to imagine that one's head is being suspended by a string from above. *The Song of the Thirteen Postures* said: "Holding the head as if suspended by a string from above, the entire body will feel light and nimble".

95

II. *The Depressing of the Chest and the Lifting of the Back*

To depress the chest is to allow the diaphragm to be lowered. This will help the intrinsic energy to sink into the "tan-tien". To lift the back is to enable the vertebrae to be vertically straight so that the strength can be effectively delivered from the spine.

III. *The Loosening of the Waist and the Drooping of the Buttocks*

The idea of loosening the waist is to make the waist light and relaxed. In Tai Chi Ch'uan all the turnings and shiftings of the body weight are controlled by the waist. *The Song of the Thirteen Postures* said: "The source of command for all movements lies in the waist". If one's waist is at ease and relaxed, not only can one's intrinsic energy easily sink into the "tan-tien" and flow freely and actively, but the lower part of the body can become strengthened, and one avoids the mistake of having the upper part heavy and the lower part light. To droop the buttocks is to allow the buttocks to sink vertically so that they do not protrude. Particularly when one squats one should pay special attention not to violate these rules. The failure of drooping the buttocks is a hindrance to the loosening of one's waist.

IV. *The Slumping of the Shoulders and the Sinking of the Elbows*

If the shoulders are not slumped the body from the chest up will be obstructed and the intrinsic energy will flow upward in an adverse manner. If the elbows are not sunk the strength cannot be increased and the hips will lose their protection.

These four points stress natural postures of the body structure of the practitioner and avoiding any unnatural uses or postures of the body. Their purpose is to allow the entire body to be completely loosened so that it can move lightly and nimbly and act in the way that one wills it to.

The Mental Aspect

V. *Directing the Movement by Using the Will*

To apply force rather than will is the number one taboo in Tai Chi Ch'uan. In all movements one should use will to direct the movements as well as to link them together. For instance, when both one's hands are moving up they are not moving up automatically by themselves, but one's will is lifting them upward. When the movement of one's will continues, the movement of one's hands continues. Once one's will discontinues, the movement of one's hands discontinues. After a long period of practice one will naturally cultivate a kind of mental power, which the Tai Chi Treatise describes as being able "To move the intrinsic energy with the mind and to permeate the body with the intrinsic energy". This is the secret of "mind over body". If beginners can comprehend the truth in this theory and manage to avoid the application of force, they will find it easier to learn the exercise and will not easily get tired of it, although the path to learning it appears simple and tasteless.

VI. *The Unification of the Form and Spirit*

The ultimate objective of Tai Chi Ch'uan practice is the cultivation of one's spirit. Therefore, while practicing the exercise one must lift one's spirit so that the spirit is in harmony with the entire body movement. Only thus can one's body be alert in responding to external stimuli and only thus can one's movement be light and nimble.

Tai Chi — "Wonderful Hand"

Chang Cheung-hsing's "Message of His Discovery of the General Theory of Tai Chi Ch'uan".

Totally Yin without Yang is "Soft Hand".

Totally Yang without Yin is "Hard Hand".

10% Yin with 90% Yang is "Hard Rod Hand".

20% Yin with 80% Yang is "Combat Hand".

30% Yin with 70% Yang results in "Rigid Hand".

40% Yin with 60% Yang may be classified as "Good Hand".

Only 50% Yang beautifully matched with 50% Yin — without being partial to either Yin or Yang — is regarded as "Wonderful Hand". The execution of "Wonderful Hand" is an expression of Tai Chi. When all images and forms are completely neutralized, things once again return to their original state of "nothingness".

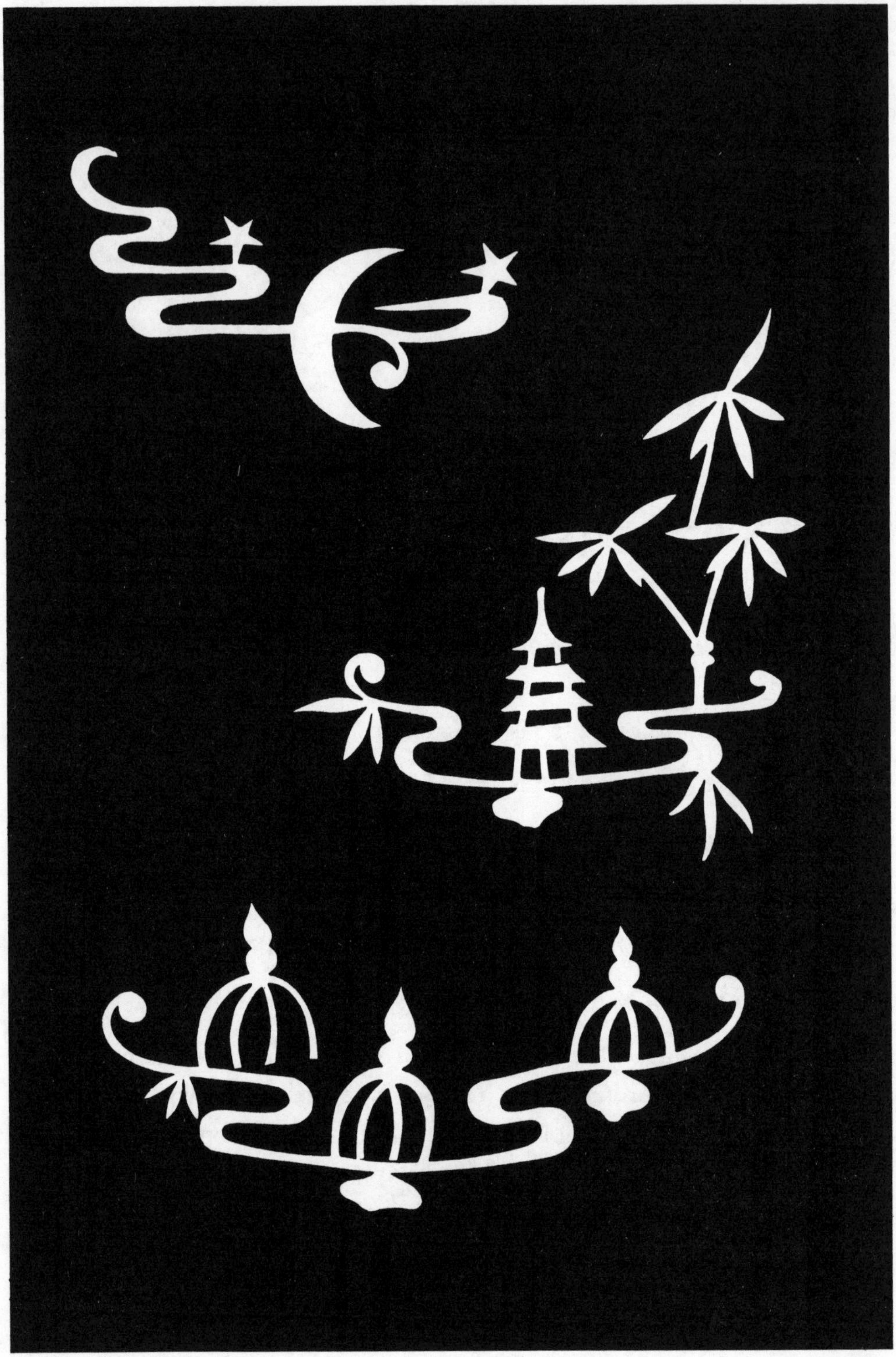

The Taoist Masters and the "I Ching"

Much of Tai Chi is completely inexplicable without reference to the intellectual and spiritual tradition of which it is a part. This is particularly true if Tai Chi is thought of as being more than just a sophisticated system of calisthentics. The primary intent of this section is to give some sense of what the Taoist tradition and the *I Ching* are about; to present a sampling of these texts which hopefully will prove to be enticing; and to explain some of the connections between Tai Chi and these philosophies.

We should point out that many Tai Chi instructors are not familiar to any great extent with these texts. Some of them are men who come out of a boxing tradition, men who spent their early years practicing more aggressive martial arts and who had little interest in the softer style and more philosophical orientation of Tai Chi. Due to age, and to a large market in this country for Tai Chi, some of these men have begun teaching the exercise. To

101

some extent the interest in Tai Chi as a martial art com-
petes with the philosophy behind the exercise. In many
schools Tai Chi is taught with an emphasis on fighting
and there is organized competition with winners and
losers. The inclinations of our teacher have led us away
from this aspect of Tai Chi. It is always enlightening,
and certainly entertaining, to see how far the human de-
viates from the theoretical. Many of the most respected
masters of Tai Chi, the art of peace, are quite contentious,
involving themselves constantly in contests of strength
and territorial challenges. Perhaps most surprising of
all is the fact that many modern day Chinese, overly
impressed with Western science and education, are anx-
ious to ignore these murky and mystical texts. In the
West, the generation of which we are a part has a greater
interest in these arcane "sciences", and is more open to
their implications.

There is no way of getting around the fact that the
texts are difficult. The first few times you read them they
may seem obscure and incomprehensible, although usually there are a few gems that everyone finds even on a
first reading. Our experience with these books, as well
as with Tai Chi, is that they must be gone over repeatedly,
not with any sense of trying to figure them out, or to
"really get them down", but with patience and a sense
of leisure. Approached in this way, passages that you
have read dozens of times will suddenly become crystal
clear — lucid confirmations of your own experience.

102

We have included sections on Lao Tzu, the principal figure in "Philosophical Taoism"; Chuang Tzu, the "enfant terrible" of Taoism; and the *I Ching*. There are essays preceding excerpts from these works which are intended as general introductions from the perspective of their relevance to Tai Chi. We have also included opiniated bibliographies for those who want to delve more deeply.

LAO TZU, THE "TAO TE CHING", AND TAI CHI

The *Tao Te Ching* by Lao Tzu, which is only 5,000 characters in length in the original Chinese, is at once a sourcebook on the mystical and spiritual life and a practical guide to survival in the world. For readers from East and West it is also a lyrical work filled with genuine insight into life.

Lao Tzu — "Old Man" in Chinese — was a contemporary of Confucius, which places him in the sixth century B.C. These dates, however, are disputed by scholars, as is in fact the very existence of the historical figure of Lao Tzu. All of the arguments one way or the other seem inconclusive. The reigning myth would have it that Lao Tzu was the official historian in charge of the archives at Chou, and that he met with Confucius, whom he chastised for his vanity, ambition, arrogance, lustfulness, and ingratiating manners. Confucius is reported to have responded to this censure by extolling Lao Tzu in the following words:

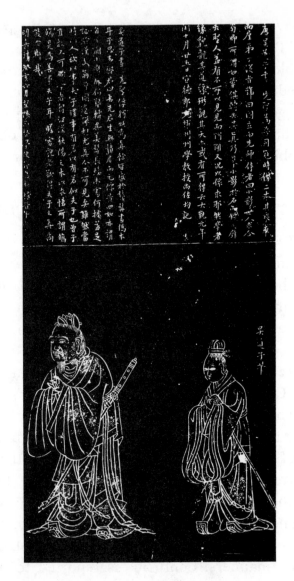

Confucius and disciple, by Wu Tao-tzu, 1107 A.D.
Courtesy of Field Museum of Natural History, Chicago.

I know a bird can fly, a fish can swim, and an animal can run. For that which runs a net can be made; for that which swims a line can be made; for that which flies a corded arrow can be made. But the dragon's ascent into heaven on the wind and clouds is something beyond my knowledge. Today I have seen Lao Tzu who is perhaps like a dragon.

So the Taoists would have it.

Seeing the decline of the Chou Dynasty, Lao Tzu felt that his time had come to retire from the active life to the obscurity of the Western mountains. But when he reached the pass leading into the wilderness, the Keeper of the Pass persuaded him to explain the "Way" and "Virtue". Lao Tzu remained there long enough to complete the two books comprising the *Tao Te Ching, (The Book of the Way and Virtue)*.

The Tao, or the Way, is all that is natural, eternal, nameless, spontaneous. The Way is filled with joyousness, and is free of fear and all that is oppressive of man's spirit. Tao is a name for what happens, or in Lao Tzu's words, for what "happens of itself". The Tao is on the one hand the realm of mystery and revelation in which man has a direct and immediate perception of the under-lying workings of the universe; and on the other hand it is our everyday life in which we loaf around, daydream, work, get drunk, fight, and make love. There is, according to Lao Tzu, no contradiction between these two worlds; both are real and significant. This is not a system in which

105

the "do-gooders" are rewarded and the idlers punished. What is asked of people is only that they not interfere with the process of life. The Taoist experiences the world with open eyes and open ears and sees what is there without reference to any past or future time . . . without asking what the moment has in it for him.

The emphasis in Lao Tzu is not on correct belief, but rather on the truth of experience. Never fight with the world because it doesn't correspond to your expectations and preconceptions. Accept what is, and learn to master it by yielding to it. Fighting what cannot be changed is responsible for much of the tragi-comedy of life. On a personal level Taoism is not a philosophy of *compelling* oneself to be calm and dignified under all circumstances. "The real and astonishing calm of people like Lao Tzu comes from the fact that they are ready and willing, without shame, to do whatever comes naturally in all circumstances" (Alan Watts).

Lao Tzu's concept of "wu-wei", or non-action, is emphatically not one of passiveness or withdrawal from the world. People live their separate lives as generals, butchers, kings, philosophers, and hermits; power and ease are granted to those who act in accord with the Tao — to those who do nothing until they have to, and then act with all of the power that comes from necessity, equilibrium, stillness, and deliberation. Ambition, greed, and the lifeless repetition of social gestures all require great

106

expenditures of energy, create fear and anxiety, and ultimately divide us against ourselves.

Relating this to Tai Chi, those who practice the art with an eye to the external signs of success rarely have the patience to succeed. Success comes more readily to those who can practice Tai Chi with the intention of enjoying the movements and the time set aside in which to "play the Tai Chi". Lao Tzu is very much the spiritual foundation of Tai Chi, guiding us to the way in which Tai Chi should be practiced, and offering insights into the physical aspects as well. Stressed are those principles which lead to suppleness, endurance, softness, centeredness, and longevity. Thus, the images of the bow which bends without breaking, the baby who is soft and durable, water which yields, flows continuously, and overcomes the hardest opponent, plants which are soft and tender, and the Sage who works without doing and knows what is "enough". For those who follow the "Way" of Tai Chi there is a growing ease and softness in movement, and finally the development of real and enduring strength.

A NOTE ON SOURCES

There are an enormous number of translations of the *Tao Te Ching*. Gia Fu Feng's translation is to my mind one of the most coherent and closest in spirit to Tai Chi.

Tai Chi Ch'uan

For books on Lao Tzu and Taoism I recommend *The Way and Its Power: A Study of the "Tao Te Ching" and Its Place in Chinese Thought* by Arthur Waley, Grove Press, 1958. *Taoism: The Way of the Mystic* by J. C. Cooper, Samuel Weiser, 1972 is quite good. *Lao Tzu and Taoism* by Max Kaltenmark, Stanford, 1969 and *Tao: The Watercourse Way* by Alan Watts, Pantheon, 1975 are worthwhile. Finally, for those interested in a good introduction to Chinese philosophy I highly recommend *A Source Book in Chinese Philosophy* translated and compiled by Wing-Tsit Chan, Princeton, 1963. All of these books are available in paperback editions.

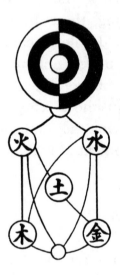

A diagram of the Grand Terminus designed by Chou Lien-chi, a noted metaphysician of the Sung Dynasty (1017–1073 A.D.).

108

SELECTIONS FROM THE "TAO TE CHING"

EIGHT

The highest good is like water.
Water gives life to the ten thousand things and does not strive.
It flows in places men reject and so is like the Tao.

In dwelling, be close to the land.
In meditation, go deep in the heart.
In dealing with others, be gentle and kind.
In speech, be true.
In ruling, be just.
In business, be competent.
In action, watch the timing.

No fight: No blame.

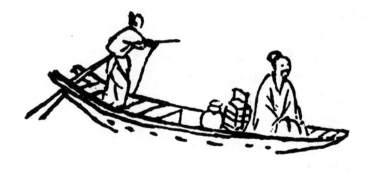

From the *Mustard Seed Garden Manual*.

Tai Chi Ch'uan

NINE

Better stop short than fill to the brim.
Oversharpen the blade, and the edge will soon blunt.
Amass a store of gold and jade, and no one can protect it.
Claim wealth and titles, and disaster will follow.
Retire when the work is done.
This is the way of heaven.

TEN

Carrying body and soul and embracing the one.
Can you avoid separation?
Attending fully and becoming supple,
Can you be as a newborn babe?
Washing and cleansing the primal vision.
Can you be without stain?
Loving all men and ruling the country.
Can you be without cleverness?
Opening and closing the gates of heaven.
Can you play the role of woman?
Understanding and being open to all things,
Are you able to do nothing?
Giving birth and nourishing,
Bearing yet not possessing,
Working yet not taking credit,
Leading yet not dominating,
This is the Primal Virtue.

FIFTEEN

The ancient masters were subtle, mysterious, profound,
    responsive.
The depth of their knowledge is unfathomable.
Because it is unfathomable,
All we can do is describe their appearance.
Watchful, like men crossing a winter stream.
Alert, like men aware of danger.
Courteous, like visiting guests.
Yielding, like ice about to melt.
Simple, like uncarved blocks of wood.
Hollow, like caves.
Opaque, like muddy pools.

Who can wait quietly while the mud settles?
Who can remain still until the moment of action?
Observers of the Tao do not seek fulfillment.
Not seeking fulfillment, they are not swayed by desire for change.

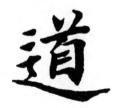

The Chinese character for Tao, translated as The Way, the path, the standard.

111

Tai Chi Ch'uan

EIGHTEEN

When the great Tao is forgotten,
Kindness and morality arise.
When wisdom and intelligence are born,
The great pretense begins.

When there is no peace within the family,
Filial piety and devotion arise.
When the country is confused and in chaos,
Loyal ministers appear.

NINETEEN

Give up sainthood, renounce wisdom,
And it will be a hundred times better for everyone.

Give up kindness, renounce morality,
And men will rediscover filial piety and love.

Give up ingenuity, renounce profit,
And bandits and thieves will disappear.

These three are outward forms alone; they are not sufficient
    in themselves.
It is more important
To see the simplicity,
To realize one's true nature,

To cast off selfishness
And temper desire.

TWENTY-TWO

Yield and overcome;
Bend and be straight;
Empty and be full;
Wear out and be new;
Have little and gain;
Have much and be confused.

Therefore wise men embrace the one
And set an example to all.
Not putting on a display,
They shine forth.
Not justifying themselves.
They are distinguished.
Not boasting,
They receive recognition.
Not bragging,
They never falter.
They do not quarrel,
So no one quarrels with them.
Therefore the ancients say, "Yield and overcome".
Is that an empty saying?
Be really whole,
And all things will come to you.

Tai Chi Ch'uan

TWENTY FOUR

He who stands on tiptoe is not steady.
He who strides cannot maintain the pace.
He who makes a show is not enlightened.
He who is self-righteous is not respected.
He who boasts achieves nothing.
He who brags will not endure.
According to followers of the Tao,
    "These are extra food and unnecessary luggage."
They do not bring happiness.
Therefore followers of the Tao avoid them.

THIRTY-THREE

Knowing others is wisdom;
Knowing the self is enlightenment.
Mastering others requires force;
Mastering the self needs strength.

He who knows he has enough is rich.
Perseverance is a sign of will power.
He who stays where he is endures.
To die but not to perish is to be eternally present.

The Taoist Masters and the "I Ching"

FORTY-THREE

The softest thing in the universe
Overcomes the hardest thing in the universe.
That without substance can enter where there is no room.
Hence I know the value of non-action.

Teaching without words and work without doing
Are understood by very few.

FORTY-SEVEN

Without going outside, you may know the whole world.
Without looking through the window,
    you may see the ways of heaven.
The farther you go, the less you know.

Thus the sage knows without traveling;
He sees without looking;
He works without doing.

FORTY-EIGHT

In the pursuit of learning, every day something is acquired.
In the pursuit of Tao, every day something is dropped.

Tai Chi Ch'uan

Less and less is done.
Until non-action is achieved.
When nothing is done, nothing is left undone.

The world is ruled by letting things take their course.
It cannot be ruled by interfering.

FIFTY-FIVE

He who is filled with Virtue is like a newborn child.
Wasps and serpents will not sting him;
Wild beasts will not pounce upon him;
He will not be attacked by birds of prey.
His bones are soft, his muscles weak,
But his grip is firm.
He has not experienced the union of man and woman,
    but is whole.
His manhood is strong.
He screams all day without becoming hoarse.
This is perfect harmony.

Knowing harmony is constancy.
Knowing constancy is enlightenment.

It is not wise to rush about.
Controlling the breath causes strain.
If too much energy is used, exhaustion follows.

116

This is not the way of Tao.
Whatever is contrary to Tao will not last long.

SIXTY-THREE

Practice non-action.
Work without doing.
Taste the tasteless.
Magnify the small, increase the few.
Reward bitterness with care.

See simplicity in the complicated.
Achieve greatness in little things.

In the universe the difficult things are done as if they are easy.
In the universe great acts are made up of small deeds.
The sage does not attempt anything very big.
And thus achieves greatness.

Easy promises make for little trust.
Taking things lightly results in great difficulty.
Because the sage always confronts difficulties,
He never experiences them.

Wu Wei or non-action.　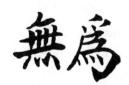

Tai Chi Ch'uan

SIXTY-NINE

There is a saying among soldiers:
    I dare not make the first move
        but would rather play the guest;
    I dare not advance an inch
        but would rather withdraw a foot.

This is called marching without appearing to move,
Rolling up your sleeves without showing your arm,
Capturing the enemy without attacking.
Being armed without weapons.

There is no greater catastrophe than underestimating the enemy.
By underestimating the enemy, I almost lose what I value.

Therefore when the battle is joined,
The underdog will win.

SIXTY-EIGHT

A good soldier is not violent.
A good fighter is not angry.
A good winner is not vengeful.
A good employer is humble.
This is known as the Virtue of not striving.
This is known as ability to deal with people.
This since ancient times has been known
    as the ultimate unity with heaven.

118

SEVENTY-SEVEN

The Tao of heaven is like the bending of a bow.
The high is lowered, and the low is raised.
If the string is too long, it is shortened;
If there is not enough, it is made longer.

The Tao of heaven is to take from those who have too much
    and give to those who do not have enough.
Man's way is different.
He takes from those who do not have enough
    to give to those who already have too much.
What man has more than enough and gives it to the world?
Only the man of Tao.

Therefore the sage works without recognition.
He achieves what has to done without dwelling on it.
He does not try to show his knowledge.

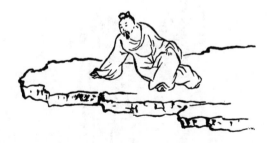

From the *Chieh Tzu Yuan Hua Chuan, Mustard Seed Garden Manual of Painting*, a seventeenth century text on painting. This illustration is "Lying on a rock flat as a mat, head bent, watching the long flowing stream".

Tai Chi Ch'uan

SEVENTY-SIX

A man is born gentle and weak.
At his death he is hard and stiff.
Green plants are tender and filled with sap.
At their death they are withered and dry.

Therefore the stiff and unbending is the disciple of death.
The gentle and yielding is the disciple of life.

Thus an army without flexibility never wins a battle.
A tree that is unbending is easily broken.

The hard and strong will fall.
The soft and weak will overcome.

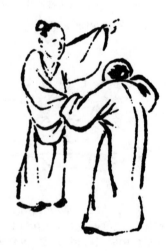

From "The Book of People and Things" from the *Mustard Seed Garden Manual*.

CHUANG TZU

Chuang Tzu is a delightful philosopher — bright, irreverent, and wise. Where Lao Tzu is somewhat detached, Chuang Tzu is vigorous and filled with earthy humor. He instructs his readers however he can: charming them, persuading them with logic, shocking them with absurdities.

Chuang Tzu excels as a story teller, and his writings abound with wonderful characters: the man who was so ugly that you couldn't bear to look at him, but so good that in the end you couldn't help but love him; a wild man filled with the Tao who spent his days joyously slapping his buttocks; and a ponderous, pretentious, slightly out-of-focus Confucius.

Like any great philosopher Chuang Tzu goes right to the heart of things with the questions that he asks. What is life? How should we lead our lives? Frequently he answers his own questions by way of negative examples of foolishness and human waste. He has a particular axe to grind with those who transgress against the laws of life in the name of goodness and virtue. What difference is there, he asks, between the robber killed while thieving and the martyr who throws down his life in the name of a cause? Both have thrown their lives away. This is a central concern — how do people come to throw away life in the name of an *idea* of right and wrong? Seeing the world through rigid and immutable categories is a folly which frequently results in tragedy.

This is a very radical statement which one is inclined to dismiss as hyperbole, or to view as an attack on the Confucian obsession with proper conduct. Both of these elements are probably there, but I believe that Chuang Tzu is to be taken at his word, and that what is strongest and most unique in his philosophy comes from this curiously amoral perception. It is easy to see the errors of murderers and thieves, but harder to see what it is about "good" men which leads them to unhappiness and often futile death.

The trap for those who are overly concerned with being "good" is that "the good" becomes more and more remote from their lives as they become prisoners of their *thoughts* about the world; spontaneous action, creativity, and the immediate experience of life are lost. To truly understand life it is necessary to experience it, to go directly to things themselves. Chuang Tzu's criticism of society here is relevant and seems remarkably contemporaneous. All of us can see, can hear, can think. Why do we allow ourselves to become convinced that we can't, that we must rely on a few select experts or professionals? They can really hear, but we can't. They can really think, but we can't. They could really know what was going on in Vietnam, but we couldn't. Nonsense, says Chuang Tzu, these are all things that we can do *naturally*.

Think about all of the things we were convinced we couldn't do as children, things which we have had to painfully rediscover as adults. But more than just the development of skills is at stake here. The real question is the loss of our sense of responsibility for ourselves and the world of which we are a part. In Chuang Tzu's words:

> When men possessed and employed their natural power of vision there was no distortion in the world. When they possessed and employed their natural power of hearing there was no distraction in the world. When they possessed and employed their natural faculty of knowledge there was no delusion in the world. When they possessed and employed their natural virtue there was no depravity in the world.

And the sages, and law-makers, and religious leaders are as much to blame as anyone, for they turn the perception of a moment into dogma which in turn creates an oppressive and unliveable system for all.

Chuang Tzu's heroes frequently are characters who act mindlessly and instinctively, and who in this way come to a particularized understanding of the workings of the universe and of the Tao. These characters — sometimes "fools", sometimes craftsmen, or statesmen — act neither from a desire for personal gain nor from a sense of moral obligation. The butcher involved in cutting up a carcass, the cabinet maker constructing a bell stand, they respond openly and fully to the moment of which they are a part. From them rulers, moralists, and philosophers must learn.

This is all very neat and convincing on paper. It sounds so true and wise, so familiar. You can read it and

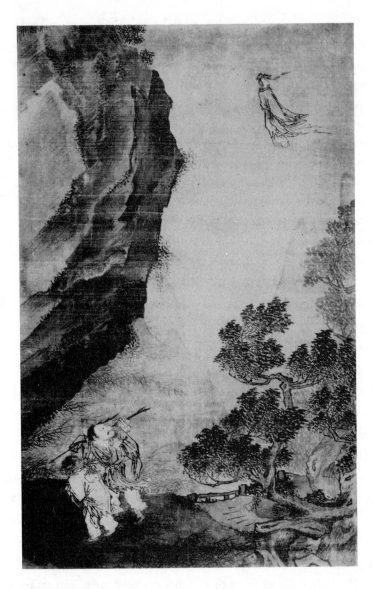

A flying Taoist Saint.
Courtesy of Field Museum of Natural History, Chicago.

have it slide right through your head. How do you hold onto it? This is the very question that Chuang Tzu asks in his parable of the wheelmaker and his sovereign. The wheelmaker, coming upon his sovereign reading, asks him why he is wasting his time with "the dregs and sediments of those old men". The duke, offended, tells the wheelwright to explain himself or die. The craftsman goes on to describe how with him the reality of making wheels doesn't exist in words or in explanations but only in the actual making of wheels. He has not been able to teach even his son how to make them properly, and so, at his advanced age, he goes on making them himself. On hearing this the duke realizes the wisdom of the remarks and spares his life. The reality of making good wheels lies not in talking about them, or in ideas about making them, but in the actual process of making the wheels. What we truly know, we know almost unconsciously, and we do effortlessly. We know how to breathe and how to walk. Some of us have highly developed skills while others of us have natural gifts like the ability to sing or to dance. These are the things that we know the best, and they are the means whereby we can be most in touch with ourselves and with the Tao. Chuang Tzu continually reminds his readers that what is important is not his words, but what lies behind them. "Words are like the waves acted on by the wind." Try to get their substance, then discard them.

And so it is with the Sage; his is not an abstract wisdom, but the concrete reality of day-to-day life. He is very human. Foolishness, pettiness, and anger are part of him, as they are part of all of us. His essence is his naturalness. He frowns when he is disturbed, laughs when happy, sleeps when tired. The Tao is there, and here, in all of this — in the sky, in the trees, in this blade of grass, even in this turd.

Rather than being set apart from men, the sage is everything that they are and more. He is the man who sits fishing by the river picking his toes, *and* the man who soars to spiritual heights. "Alone he associates with Heaven and Earth and spirit, without abandoning or desiring things of the world." His secret lies in the fact that for him fame is no better than obscurity, wealth not more to be desired than poverty, life no better than death.

Chuang Tzu's ideas are the ancestors of the spiritual disciplines that eventually became Chan Buddhism in China and Zen in Japan. They share a rejection of verbal logic and conventional morality. The road to enlightenment is an inward turning pathway leading us back to our original nature. It is a path which rejects the excesses of self-abuse, flagellation, or extreme mental or physical disciplines. It is a way marked more by laughter and joyousness than by will power and determination. An eleventh century poem by Cheng Hao captures something of this spirit.

Near the middle of the day, when clouds are thin and
  breeze soft,
I stroll beside the river, passing the willows and the
  trees in bloom.
People of the day do not understand my joy;
They say that I am loafing like an idle young man.

Scattered throughout Chuang Tzu's writing is a good
deal of information relating to the body, all of which is in
conformity with the principles of Tai Chi. There is a belief that we have within us a power that is most successfully expressed in "natural" forms of movement. The perfect example of this is the baby who in Chuang Tzu's tale
can keep its fist clenched all day long and shout from
morning until evening without tiring. This is because the
baby's spirit is entire and concentrated. He is a natural
and conscious version of the drunk who falls from a car-
riage and remains unhurt because his spirit is entire and
his body indifferent. Chuang Tzu is critical of those who
practice extreme forms of exercise — the fourth century
B.C. version of the Canadian Air Force Exercises.
  What is known of Chuang Tzu himself is extremely
limited. According to the earliest accounts of him, he
lived in Meng and served as an official in the "Lacquer
Garden" sometime in the fourth century B.C. His work is
divided into three parts: the seven "Inner Chapters"
which are considered to be the basic body of his work,
fifteen "Outer Chapters" thought to be more adulterated,

and eleven "Miscellaneous Chapters". Our selections are from all three sections.

A NOTE ON SOURCES

The translations of Chuang Tzu tend to be considerably less literate than those of Lao Tzu, and also less numerous. For complete translations we recommend *The Complete Works of Chuang Tzu* by Burton Watson, Columbia University Press, 1968. Burton Watson has also put together an abridged version which is available in paper from Columbia University Press titled *Chuang Tzu: Basic Writings*. James Legge's *The Texts of Taoism*, Dover, 1962, was originally published in 1891. The prose is good, though at times a bit ponderous. Selections from Chuang Tzu are available in Arthur Waley's *Three Ways of Thought in Ancient China*, Doubleday, 1939, and *The Way of Chuang Tzu* by Thomas Merton, New Directions, 1965. Merton, in a long introduction, relates Chuang Tzu's mysticism to similar strains in Catholicism. Finally, Gia-feu Feng and Jane English have a companion to their Lao Tzu which is attractive though not quite as comprehensible as the previous work. *Chuang Tzu: Inner Chapters*, Vintage, 1974.

SELECTIONS FROM CHUANG TZU

FREE AND EASY WANDERING

The morning mushroom knows nothing of twilight and dawn; the summer cicada knows nothing of spring and autumn. They are the short-lived. South of Ch'u there is a caterpillar which counts five hundred years as one spring and five hundred years as one autumn. Long, long ago there was a great rose of Sharon that counted eight thousand years as one spring and eight thousand years as one autumn. They are the long-lived.

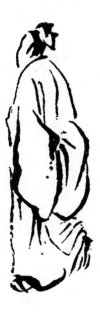

Hsieh i style of figure drawing. Translated as *write idea of grass style.* From the *Mustard Seed Garden Manual.*

Tai Chi Ch'uan

DISCUSSION ON MAKING ALL THINGS EQUAL

Great understanding is broad and unhurried; little understanding is cramped and busy. Great words are clear and limpid; little words are shrill and quarrelsome. In sleep, men's spirits go visiting; in waking hours, their bodies hustle. With everything they meet they become entangled. Day after day they use their minds in strife, sometimes grandiose, sometimes sly, sometimes petty. Their little fears are mean and trembly; their great fears are stunned and overwhelming. They bound off like an arrow or a crossbow pellet, certain that they are the arbiters of right and wrong. They cling to their position as though they had sworn before the gods, sure that they are holding on to victory. They fade like fall and winter — such is the way they dwindle day by day. They drown in what they do — you cannot make them turn back. They grow dark, as though sealed with seals — such are the excesses of their old age. And when their minds draw near to death, nothing can restore them to the light.

*   *   *

But to wear out your brain trying to make things into one without realizing that they are all the same — this is called "three in the morning". What do I mean by "three in the morning"? When the monkey trainer was handing out acorns, he said, "You get three in the morning and four at night". This made all the monkeys furious. "Well, then", he said, "you get four in the morning and three at night." The monkeys were all delighted.

130

There was no change in the reality behind the words, and yet the monkeys responded with joy and anger. Let them, if they want to. So the sage harmonizes with both right and wrong and rests in Heaven the Equalizer. This is called walking two roads.

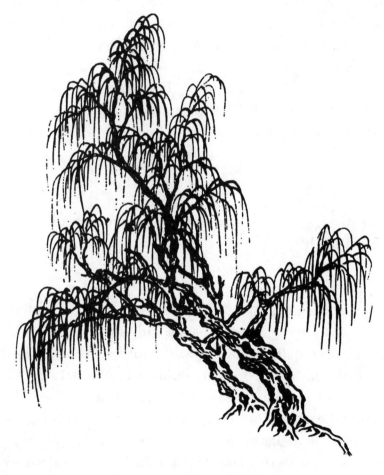

Willow tree from the *Mustard Seed Garden Manual*.

Tai Chi Ch'uan

* * *

The sage leans on the sun and moon, tucks the universe under his arm, merges himself with things, leaves the confusion and muddle as it is, and looks on slaves as exalted. Ordinary men strain and struggle; the sage is stupid and blockish. He takes part in ten thousand ages and achieves simplicity in oneness. For him, all the ten thousand things are what they are, and thus they enfold each other.

How do I know that loving life is not a delusion? How do I know that in hating death I am not like a man who having left home in his youth, has forgotten the way back?

* * *

How do I know that the dead do not wonder why they ever longed for life?

* * *

Once Chuang Chou dreamt he was a butterfly, a butterfly flitting and fluttering around, happy with himself and doing as he pleased. He didn't know he was Chuang Chou. Suddenly he woke up and there he was, solid and unmistakable Chuang Chou. But he didn't know if he was Chuang Chou who had dreamt he was a butterfly, or a butterfly dreaming he was Chuang Chou. Between Chuang Chou and a butterfly there must be *some* distinction! This is called the Transformation of Things.

132

IN THE WORLD OF MEN

The mountain trees do themselves harm; the grease in the torch burns itself up. The cinnamon can be eaten and so it gets cut down; the lacquer tree can be used and so it gets hacked apart. All men know the use of the useful, but nobody knows the use of the useless!

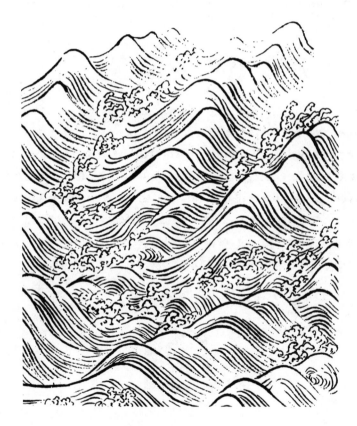

From the *Garden Seed Manual of Painting.*

Tai Chi Ch'uan

THE GREAT AND VENERABLE TEACHER

The True Man of ancient times knew nothing of loving life, knew nothing of hating death. He emerged without delight; he went back in without a fuss. He came briskly, he went briskly, and that was all. He didn't forget where he began; he didn't try to find out where he would end. He received something and took pleasure in it; he forgot about it and handed it back again.

FIT FOR EMPERORS AND KINGS

Do not be an embodier of fame; do not be a storehouse of schemes; do not be an undertaker of projects; do not be a proprietor of wisdom. Embody to the fullest what has no end and wander where there is no trail. Hold on to all that you have received from Heaven but do not think you have gotten anything. Be empty, that is all. The Perfect Man uses his mind like a mirror — going after nothing, welcoming nothing, responding but not storing. Therefore he can win out over things and not hurt himself.

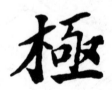

Chinese character for Chi.

134

WEBBED TOES

He who holds to True Rightness does not lose the original form of his inborn nature. So for him joined things are not webbed toes, things forking off are not superfluous fingers, the long is never too much, the short is never too little.

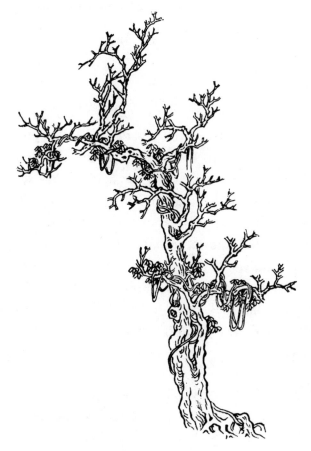

From the *Mustard Seed Garden Manual*, "The Book of Trees".

Everyone in the world risks his life for something. If he risks it for benevolence and righteousness, then custom names him a gentleman; if he risks it for goods and wealth, then custom names him a petty man. The risking is the same, and yet we have a gentleman here, a petty man there. In destroying their lives and blighting their inborn nature, Robber Chih and Po Yi were two of a kind. How then can we pick out the gentleman from the petty man in such a case?

HEAVEN AND EARTH

In an age of Perfect Virtue the worthy are not honored, the talented are not employed. Rulers are like the high branches of a tree, the people like the deer of the fields. They do what is right but they do not know that this is righteousness. They love one another but they do not know that this is benevolence. They are truehearted but do not know that this is loyalty. They are trustworthy but do not know that this is good faith. They wriggle around like insects, performing services for one another but do not know that they are being kind. Therefore they move without leaving any trail behind, act without leaving any memory of their deeds.

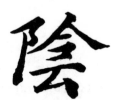

The Chinese character for Yin.

THE TURNING OF HEAVEN

Rituals and regulations are something that change in response to the times.

AUTUMN FLOODS

There is no end to the weighing of things, no stop to time, no constancy to the division of lots, no fixed rules to beginning and end. Therefore great wisdom observes both far and near, and for that reason recognizes small without considering it paltry, recognizes large without considering it unwieldy, for it knows that there is no end to the weighing of things. It has a clear understanding of past and present, and for that reason it spends a long time without finding it tedious, a short time without fretting at its shortness, for it knows that time has no stop. It perceives the nature of fullness and emptiness, and for that reason it does not delight if it acquires something nor worry if it loses it, for it knows that there is no constancy to the division of lots. It comprehends the Level Road, and for that reason it does not rejoice in life nor look on death as a calamity, for it knows that no fixed rule can be assigned to beginning and end.

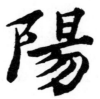

The Chinese character for Yang.

Tai Chi Ch'uan

*   *   *

The Way is without beginning or end, but things have their life and death — you cannot rely upon their fulfillment. One moment empty, the next moment full — you cannot depend upon their form. The years cannot be held off; time cannot be stopped. Decay, growth, fullness, and emptiness end and then begin again. It is thus that we must describe the plan of the Great Meaning and discuss the principles of the ten thousand things. The life of things is a gallop, a headlong dash — with every movement they alter, with every moment they shift. What should you do and what should you not do? Everything will change of itself, that is certain!

*   *   *

Once, when Chuang Tzu was fishing in the P'u River, the king of Ch'u sent two officials to go and announce to him: "I would like to trouble you with the administration of my realm."

Chuang Tzu held on to the fishing pole and, without turning his head, said, "I have heard that there is a sacred tortoise in Ch'u that has been dead for three thousand years. The king keeps it wrapped in cloth and boxed, and stores it in the ancestral temple. Now would this tortoise rather be dead and have its bones left behind and honored? Or would it rather be alive and dragging its tail in the mud?"

"It would rather be alive and dragging its tail in the mud," said the two officials.

Chuang Tzu said, "Go away! I'll drag my tail in the mud!"

138

The Taoist Masters and the "I Ching"

* * *

Chuang Tzu and Hui Tzu were strolling along the dam of the Hao River when Chuang Tzu said, "See how the minnows come out and dart around where they please! That's what fish really enjoy!"

Hui Tzu said, "You're not a fish — how do you know what fish enjoy?"

Chuang Tzu said, "You're not I, so how do you know I don't know what fish enjoy?"

Tui Tzu said, "I'm not you, so I certainly don't know what you know. On the other hand, you're certainly not a fish — so that still proves you don't know what fish enjoy!"

Chuang Tzu said, "Let's go back to your original question, please. You asked me *how* I know what fish enjoy — so you already knew I knew it when you asked the question. I know it by standing here beside the Hao".

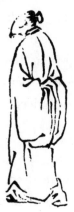

"Walking in autumn, with hands clasped behind." From the seventeenth century *Mustard Seed Garden Manual.*

139

Tai Chi Ch'uan

PERFECT HAPPINESS

This is what the world honors: wealth, eminence, long life, a good name. This is what the world finds happiness in: a life of ease, rich food, fine clothes, beautiful sights, sweet sounds. This is what it looks down on: poverty, meanness, early death, a bad name. This is what it finds bitter: a life that knows no rest, a mouth that gets no rich food, no fine clothes for the body, no beautiful sights for the eye, no sweet sounds for the ear.

*   *   *

People who can't get these things fret a great deal and are afraid — this is a stupid way to treat the body. People who are rich wear themselves out rushing around on business, piling up more wealth than they could ever use — this is a superficial way to treat the body. People who are eminent spend night and day scheming and wondering if they are doing right — this is a shoddy way to treat the body. Man lives his life in company with worry, and if he lives a long while, till he's dull and doddering, then he has spent that much time worrying instead of dying, a bitter lot indeed! This is a callous way to treat the body.

*   *   *

Chuang Tzu's wife died. When Hui Tzu went to convey his condolences, he found Chuang Tzu sitting with his legs sprawled out, pounding on a tub and singing. "You lived with her, she brought up your children and grew old," said Hui Tzu. "It

140

should be enough simply not to weep at her death. But pounding on a tub and singing — this is going too far, isn't it?"

Chuang Tzu said, "You're wrong. When she first died, do you think I didn't grieve like anyone else? But I looked back to her beginning and the time before she was born. Not only the time before she was born, but the time before she had a body. Not only the time before she had a body, but the time before she had a spirit. In the midst of the jumble of wonder and mystery a change took place and she had a spirit. Another change and she had a body. Another change and she was born. Now there's been another change and she's dead. It's just like the progression of the four seasons, spring, summer, fall, winter.

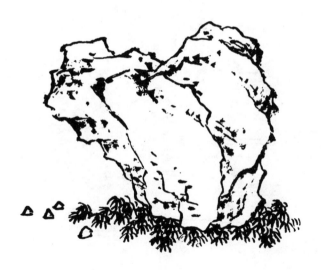

From "The Book of Rocks" from the seventeenth century *Mustard Seed Garden Manual of Painting.*

"Now she's going to lie down peacefully in a vast room. If I were to follow after her bawling and sobbing, it would show that I don't understand anything about fate. So I stopped."

*   *   *

Fish live in water and thrive, but if men tried to live in water they would die. Creatures differ because they have different likes and dislikes. Therefore the former sages never required the same ability from all creatures or made them all do the same thing. Names should stop when they have expressed reality,

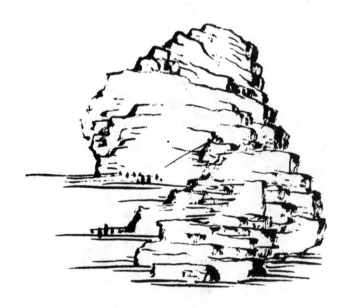

From "The Book of Rocks" of the *Mustard Seed Garden Manual of Painting*. Iron Band Brushstroke Style.

concepts of right should be founded on what is suitable. This is what it means to have command of reason, and good fortune to support you.

MASTERING LIFE

Woodworker Ch'ing carved a piece of wood and made a bell stand, and when it was finished, everyone who saw it marveled, for it seemed to be the work of gods or spirits. When the marquis of Lu saw it, he asked, "What art is it you have?"

Ch'ing replied, "I am only a craftsman — how would I have any art? There is one thing, however. When I am going to make a bell stand, I never let it wear out my energy. I always fast in order to still my mind. When I have fasted for three days, I no longer have any thought of congratulations or rewards, of titles or stipends. When I have fasted for five days, I no longer have any thought of praise or blame, of skill or clumsiness. And when I have fasted for seven days, I am so still that I forget I have four limbs and a form and body. By that time, the ruler and his court no longer exist for me. My skill is concentrated and all outside distractions fade away. After that, I go into the mountain forest and examine the Heavenly nature of the trees. If I find one of superlative form, and I can see a bell stand there, I put my hand to the job of carving; if not, I let it go. This way I am simply matching up "Heaven" with "Heaven". That's probably the reason that people wonder if the results were not made by spirits."

143

THE "I CHING" OR "THE BOOK OF CHANGES"

The *I Ching,* or *Book of Changes,* is a literary oracle — a book which can be engaged in dialogue. Like any oracle, it is a response to the basic and continuing need to make sense of our lives, to understand how and why things happen, and to find stable guidelines for our actions. It is an effort to gain control in times of confusion, even though the process seemingly involves relinquishing this control and asking an outside source what we are to do.

The text is full of ambiguities, especially for Western readers, and is not clearly understood even by scholars fluent in Chinese who have devoted their lives to its study. To consult the book, you concentrate on a specific question. By means of a carefully prescribed chance operation (tossing three coins is the most common method) you locate the "answer". This is not a simple yes or no, but a series of images, more or less obscure and suggestive. We must suspend our demand for easy answers, and allow the images to reverberate. Gradually we clarify our confusion of guilt and desire, fear and ambition. The book deals with a vast spectrum of human possibilities: Peace, Conflict, Fellowship, Youthful Folly, Enthusiasm, Splitting Apart, Oppression, Inner Truth. The answers deal with life on the levels of the social, the political, the family, and the individual.

The phenomenon of change is the obvious point at which to start thinking about the *I Ching.* In the *I Ching* change is always conceived of as a part, or a phase, of a complete cycle. The seed, for instance, is the first step in a process of development that ultimately results in the full grown tree. An understanding of this process enables us to go back to the beginnings of the situation, to the seed, or to project into the future and to see the full grown tree. Change is not random and sporadic and external, but a clearly defined process of internal evolution, even though we may not always be able to discern the pattern. How rational and scientific this seems in contrast to the kind of change or fate decreed by the whimsical, often cruel, God of the Old Testament, or the capricious, petty gods of the Greeks.

Another good image of change is the river which flows on continuously. Caught in the flow we as individuals have a number of options. We can struggle against the current, or we can float with the current, and direct our movements to either shore. In troubled waters we must be more attentive, in calm waters we can be more relaxed. But within the constraints imposed on us by the river, we choose what to do. We can choose to continually fight the current, perhaps because we want to go back to where we came from, or we can accept the fact that we are traveling into new territory.

Judgments are made in the *I Ching* about how we should deal with the flow of events. This is an oracle with a point of view — a perspective of genuine depth and complexity. One character, called the "Superior Man", is the moral hero of the *I Ching*. He makes the best of every situation. He masters fate and change by accepting it. He is equally at home leading a quiet, reflective life or being an aggressive decisive leader. He is flexible enough to mold himself to the requirements of the times. The emphasis, however, is on finding inner peace by being in harmony with life. Fame, fortune, and success are just one part of a cycle which includes obscurity, poverty, and failure. These are only to a limited degree under our control. The "Superior Man" understands this, and accepts what life deals him.

Embedded in the very structure of the book is a sense of seasonal change, change that is regular and returns to the same point. The cycles are a reassurance that things will change when times are bad, or when life is fallow, and a warning that times of plenty, prosperity, and sunshine too are only a phase of the cycle.

The *I Ching* also embodies a particular conception of human nature. It assumes, skeptically, that most of us do things for reasons of which we are only dimly aware. Great emphasis is placed on analyzing our motives, rethinking what we are doing and why we are doing it, distinguishing between what we are and are not responsible for, and finally, acting.

* * *

The basic units of the readings in the *I Ching* are the Lines, which originated in a time of pre-history with a character named Fu Hsi. The lines are of two kinds; the Yin line which is broken ___ ___ and the Yang line which is unbroken _____.

The easiest method of consulting the oracle is to toss three coins six times. Heads gives you the number two, tails gives you the number three. For each toss you add up the heads and tails of the three coins. If you get, let us say, two tails and a head, your sum is eight. The possible sums include six, seven, eight, or nine. Each of these numbers represents a Line — the even numbers give broken Yin lines; the odd numbers are unbroken Yang lines. You end up with six lines, or a hexagram, which is "read" from the bottom up. A possible hexagram looks like this —

<pre>
___ ___   6

___ ___   8

_____   7

_____   9

___ ___   6

_____   7
</pre>

Mathematically, there are sixty-four possible hexagrams, which are charted in the book. Each series of lines is a symbolic representation of the dynamic forces of change.

147

Tai Chi Ch'uan

The book developed over many centuries, and through many different traditions of thought. The original single lines were simple answers — yes or no. Eventually the Lines were combined to form pairs, and then Trigrams. Finally, the eight possible Trigrams were combined to form the Hexagrams, images of "all that happens in heaven and on earth". Traditionally, King Wên is given credit for having compiled the hexagrams in the twelfth century B.C. The Hexagram is a highly abstract rendering of the shape of change. The positive and negative lines are seen as evolving into one another, forming patterns which echo the events of our lives. When you have thrown your Hexagram, you look it up in the book and read the interpretation, or Judgment. The Judgments are credited to the Duke of Chou, son of King Wên.

King Wên and the Duke of Chou changed the nature of the oracle by insisting that in every situation there was a right and a wrong course of action. The oracle was thus changed from one which told you that you were going to win the battle or inherit a lot of money, to one which allowed for choice, for correct action, and thereby gave the person consulting the oracle an active role in his own future.

The text was amplified in the intervening centuries, and a major portion — the Commentaries — was added by Confucius and his school in the fifth and fourth centuries B.C. Finally, under the Taoist influence the terms Yin and Yang came to assume their current meanings.

This is evident in the "Great Commentary", a late addition to the *I Ching*, which reflects the dichotomies of male and female, darkness and light, hard and soft.

The operation of the oracle cannot be explained satisfactorily in any scientific sense. Our modern principle of causality has no place in this system. Rather, it is assumed that at any moment we are inextricably bound up with the totality of that instant. The hexagram that we come up with when we cast the oracle is part and parcel of that moment, and is an expression of the major forces operative at that time. What is internal to our situation is mirrored in what is external. Man is an integral part of the cosmic system and goes through the same cycles of change that can be observed in the larger whole. Though these cycles are outside of man's control, it is thought to be possible to get into direct contact with them through the *I Ching*.

The book itself becomes the "medium" through which one contacts the forces in nature, or what in some traditions would be called the spirit world. In this it is unique, for there is no intermediary required, no fortune-teller or medium — at least in principle. The authority of the information is not a function of the gifts and abilities of the person consulted, but of the wisdom of the book. In China the person consulting the book could know that he wasn't turning to the authorities of one time and place, or to one school of thought, but to a text that had been built up slowly over thousands of years with

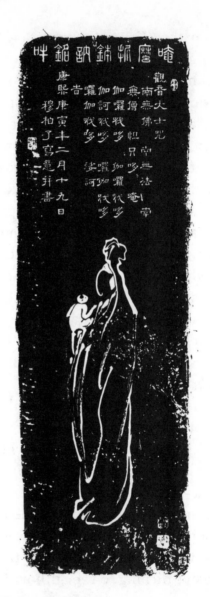

Charm of Incantation. 1710 A.D.
Courtesy of Field Museum of Natural History, Chicago.

150

inputs from innumerable people from different traditions.

In the course of writing about the *I Ching* we became interested in asking it about Tai Chi. The specific question that we asked was, "What of Tai Chi?" The hexagram that we threw was number two, K'un/The Receptive.

```
___  ___
___  ___
___  ___
___  ___
___  ___
___  ___
```

The text advised us that this hexagram represented "the dark, yielding, receptive primal power of yin". This seemed to correspond to the softness and yielding quality of Tai Chi. "It represents nature in contrast to spirit, earth in contrast to heaven, space as against time, the female-maternal as against the male-paternal."

The Judgment — which is one of the oldest sections of the book — was as follows:

> The Receptive brings about sublime success,
> Furthering through the perseverance of a mare.
> If a superior man undertakes something and tries to lead,

Tai Chi Ch'uan

> He goes astray;
> But if he follows, he finds guidance.
> It is favorable to forego friends in the east and north.
> Quiet perseverance brings good fortune.

Tai Chi is an activity which can only be approached with humility, and which is mastered by "quiet perseverance" over a long period of time. It is neither flashy nor exuberant. To undertake the study of it, it is essential to find guidance in the form of a qualified instructor, and to follow the classical texts of the discipline. To try to teach oneself, or to try to "get ahead" in the discipline leads to failure. The image of the mare is the key to all of this. In the Oriental tradition, the horse is a symbol of the earth and combines strength and swiftness with gentleness and devotion. Tai Chi is rooted in the ground with one leg always firmly planted, and combines softness and gentleness with energy and strength.

In the text — another addition to the original elements of the book — it says that "The superior man lets himself be guided. Since there is something to be accomplished, we need friends and helpers in the hour of toil and effort, once the ideas to be realized are firmly set." So it is that we learn from a teacher in the company of friends and companions. But Tai Chi is not an activity which is practiced only in a group and under supervision. The reality of Tai Chi is the solo exercise, practiced alone, where one can let the body and spirit be fully one. To this the text attests. "The East symbolizes the place where a man receives orders from his master, and the north the place where he reports on what he has done. At that minute he must be alone and objective. In this sacred hour he must do without companions, so that the purity of the moment may not be spoiled by factional hates and favoritism."

In the Commentaries this is amplified. "While the Creative shields things . . . the Receptive carries them, like a foundation that endures forever. Infinite accord with the Creative is its essence . . . The movement of the Creative is a direct forward movement, and its resting state is standstill; the movement of The Receptive is an opening out, and in its resting state it is closed. In the resting, closed state, it embraces all things as though in a vast womb. In the state of movement, of opening, it allows the divine light to enter, and by means of this light illuminates everything. This is the source of its success of living beings." Tai Chi movements are in harmony with movement in nature, and from this springs its good fortune, its strength, and endurance. In addition, it is a succession of movements which alternately open out and close in. "The good fortune of rest and perseverance depends on our being in accord with the boundless nature of the earth."

The Image — a later addition to the book which tends to give rather sophisticated interpretations of the lines — is:

> The Earth's condition is receptive devotion.
> Thus the superior man who has breadth of character
> Carries the outer world.

Just as the earth profits from its passive position and sustains life, so in Tai Chi, it is this position of receptivity and devotion that makes it possible to develop the stability and endurance necessary to carry the "outer world."

The text also includes readings for individual lines, which correspond to each line of the hexagram, and give more specific information about the situation. However, the lines are only read when you throw a six or a nine. On any one toss of the coins, if you throw three heads, or six, you have an excessively Yin line. If you throw three tails, or nine, the line is excessively Yang. Any other combination results in either a Yin or a Yang line, but ones which are not extreme. (The same theory applies to the casting of yarrow stalks, the other way of consulting the *I Ching*.)

In this casting of the *I Ching* there were three lines that were excessively Yin — the first, fourth, and fifth.

> Six at the beginning means:
> When there is hoarfrost underfoot,
> Solid ice is not far off.

"Just as the light-giving power represents life, so the

154

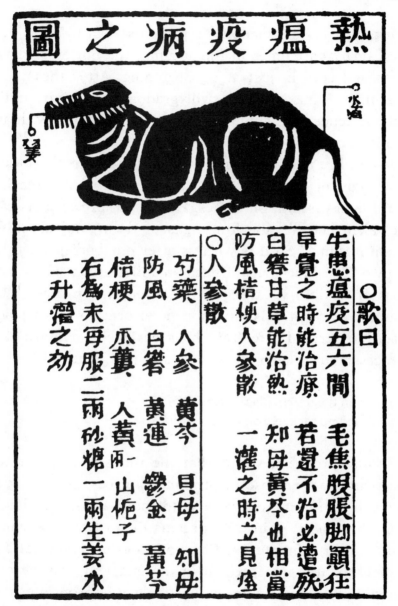

熱瘟疫病之圖

○歌曰

牛患瘟疫五六間　毛焦服脹脚顛狂
早覺之時能治療　若還不治必遭死
白礬甘草能治熱　知母黃芩也相當
防風桔梗人參散　一灌之時立見瘥

○人參散
人參　黃芩　貝母　知母
防風　白礬　黃連　鬱金　黃芩
桔梗　瓜蔞　人參兩　山恒子　黃芩
芍藥
右為末每服二兩砂糖一兩生姜水
二升灌之効

A woodcut which indicates acupuncture points used by a veterinarian.

155

dark power, the shadowy represents death. When the first hoarfrost comes in the autumn, the power of darkness and cold is just at its beginning. After these first warnings, signs of death will gradually multiply, until, in obedience to immutable laws, stark winter with its ice is here."

"In life it is the same. After certain scarcely noticeable signs of decay have appeared, they go on increasing until final dissolution comes. But in life precautions can be taken heeding the first signs of decay and checking them in time." So it is with us after our bodies are fully grown. The first signs of decay manifest themselves in a loss of flexibility, strength, and energy. For those who passively accept this situation deterioration takes place at a fairly rapid rate. Tai Chi is designed to retard this process and to keep our bodies soft and youthful.

> Six in the fourth place means:
> A tied-up sack. No blame, no praise.

The interpretation warns that the times are dangerous, particularly for those in prominent places, so that it is best to maintain reserve and to make no great claims for what one is doing. This seems like a timely warning not to over-promote Tai Chi, nor to create expectations which are too great, which in the end will only be disappointed. This warning is particulary appropriate now when the public is starved for activities that promise instant and complete change.

156

Six in the fifth place means:
A yellow lower garment brings supreme good fortune.

"yellow is the color of the earth and of the middle; it is the symbol of that which is reliable and genuine. The lower garment is inconspiculously decorated — the symbol of aristocratic reserve. A man's genuineness and refinement should not reveal themselves directly; they should express themselves only indirectly as an effect from within." The strength of Tai Chi is that it is genuine and reliable — not flashy like King Fu or acrobatics or dance. It is reserved, refined, and understated. Tai Chi is an *internal* discipline, and what is expressed on the outside is only a reflection of this internal process.

The focus of the *I Ching* is change, and even the hexagrams themselves change. All is flux. In this case all of the lines which are excessively Yin change into Yang lines, for anything that is extreme changes into its opposite. From this we derive a new hexagram, hexagram number seventeen, Sui/Following.

```
——— ———
—————————
—————————
——— ———
——— ———
—————————
```

Tai Chi Ch'uan

The second hexagram is an extension of the first situation, and its complement. In some cases it is useful to think of it as the unconscious or interior of a situation as opposed to the conscious or exterior.

The attribute of hexagram seventeen is "gladness" and the sense of it is that "Joy of movement induces following." This is exactly to the point, for this is the essence of Tai Chi, "joy in movement". The reason why people continue to do Tai Chi is in the end not because it is good for them, or because it is an interesting Oriental discipline, or because it is fashionable, but simply because it feels *good*. People continue to do it year after year because they come to love the way that it feels. And it is this quality about Tai Chi which "induces following".

The Judgment of the hexagram is that:

Following has supreme success.
Perseverance furthers. No blame.

Very much in keeping with the first hexagram.
The Image is:

Thunder in the middle of the lake:
The image of following
Thus the superior man at nightfall
Goes indoors for rest and recuperation.

The Image is of a time of darkness and rest. After exertion it is essential to rest. This applies to Tai Chi on several levels. On a day-to-day basis it is essential to have periods of time that are devoted to rest and recuperation. These take the form of sleep, and rejuvenating exercise. On a moment-to-moment basis, in the course of doing Tai Chi, there are small periods of rest that are built into the form so that after every expansion or release of energy there is a period of contraction or storing up of energy. In a larger sense, for this society in which most of us work hard and are busy much of the time, Tai Chi is a reminder that rest, recuperation, slowness, and steadiness are essential for our well-being in the long run.

In Tai Chi, and in the *I Ching*, there is no state of complete rest in the sense of stasis. There is constant motion that passes through clear and distinct points. The hexagrams are in reality only representations of "tendencies in movement", and not of fixed realities. The emphasis is on the process of moving and living. Endurance results from being in harmony with nature.

Tai Chi and the *I Ching* cannot be understood in terms of Yin or Yang, hard movements and soft, broken and unbroken lines. These are simply the "forms". "What is above form is called Tao." In Tai Chi what is beyond the physical is called "spirit". In the end Tai Chi is about the cultivation of this "spirit".

Tai Chi Ch'uan

A NOTE ON SOURCES

At this point there are a fair number of books on, and
translations of, the *I Ching*. Most of them are very peculiar. The standard, and to my mind, best translation is
still Richard Wilhelm's German translation, rendered into English by Cary Baynes. This edition includes several
useful essays by Wilhelm and C. G. Jung. *The I Ching, or
Book of Changes*, Wilhelm/Baynes, Bollingen, Princeton
University Press, 1950. Another respectable translation
with an intelligent introduction is the *I Ching, The Book
of Change* by John Blofeld, E. P. Dutton, 1968. There is a
nice collection of *Eight Lectures on the I Ching* by Hell-
mut Wilhelm, once again translated by Cary Baynes, Bollingen, Princeton University Press, 1973.

160

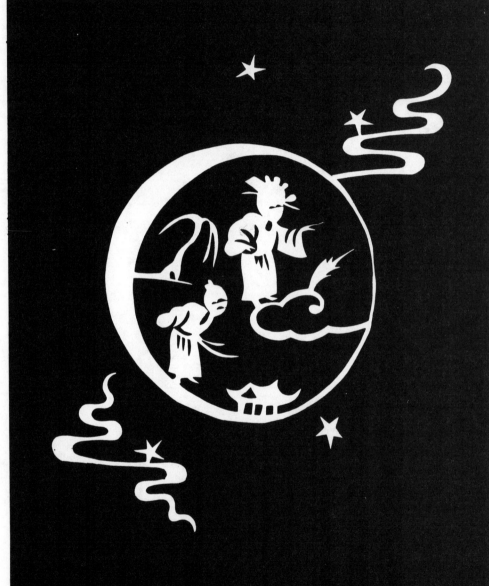

INNER WORLDS: Tai Chi, Mysticism, Magic, Meditation, and Alchemy

So much of our experience is ambiguous and subject to different interpretations. When the phone rings and it is someone you were just thinking about, is it chance, intuition, telepathy? In the case of Tai Chi, is the experience of feeling the air thicken and become like water a mystical experiencing of the world, as some would have it, or a simple physiological fact? On one level Tai Chi is merely a physical discipline — almost a calisthentic. But for those who are curious it partakes of alchemy, meditation, psychology, philosophy, even magic. Being rooted in the physical, in the body, it is solid ground from which to gaze into these murkier depths.

Mystical perceptions of the world begin with the assumption that there is something beyond our day-to-day experience of reality which is somehow more real and

163

more essential. The aim of various mystical and spiritual techniques is to penetrate behind the veil of our accustomed reality to perceive this other world. In most cultures there are individuals, traditions, or whole communities who share this perception. As many anthropologists have pointed out, there are striking similarities in descriptions of this other reality from numerous and diverse cultures. Despite the fact that there is an extensive literature dealing with this realm, the experience of it is beyond words, and is therefore incompatible with, or directly contradictory to, our conventional sense of the world. Most of us feel that we must make a choice between these two "realities"; and the choice is usually set up in such a way that we must choose between *science*, which is allied with ordinary reality, and these other traditions which we perceive as necessarily obscure, filled with superstition, and above all unmodern, perhaps the greatest sin of all. But do we in fact have to make a choice between the two? Are they really mutually exclusive options? Science is built on observation, description and method, combined with a theoretical explanation of natural phenomena. If we apply these criteria to these other activities we might be shocked to find out how fully these standards are satisfied by at least some parts of these arcane traditions. A Buddhist manual of meditation, for example, is precise, empirical, filled with psychological insight, and built on an inclusive theoretical framework. Compared to most contemporary psychology these works are masterpieces of clarity, and their conclusions and insights oddly similar to those of contemporary scientists doing basic research into the functioning of the brain. These "arcane" investigations differ from Western science not so much in method as in the phenomena investigated. It is important to remember that many mystical traditions have continuous histories that stretch back thousands of years, and that countless individuals have devoted their lives and talents to the exploration of these subjects. Is it inappropriate, then, to think of these traditions as sciences of our inner worlds?

The more serious of these inner sciences have built into them their own highly critical methods and reminders to practitioners to retain a good deal of skepticism. It is common to come across words of caution to students to take nothing for granted and to confirm all experiences personally before taking them for truth. "With these things it is just as it is when one drinks water", we read in *The Secret of the Golden Flower*, A Taoist text of meditation. "One can tell for oneself whether the water is warm or cold. In the same way a man must convince himself about these experiences, then only are they real." To step into the unknown is a risky business, these texts insist, and must be undertaken in a disciplined and methodical way. Great explorers rarely fail to make use of all the information they can obtain beforehand about where they are going, and always take great care to bring along everything they might need on the voyage. Those who explore the realms we are dealing with in this chapter necessarily have a great curiosity, one which is not satisfied by simply reading or talking about *other* people's ideas of the world.

It is no accident that the roots of modern science go back to these arcane disciplines. In the West it is easy to forget that the fathers of modern science were astrologers, alchemists, and numerologists, and that men like Newton and Galileo used science in the service of theology. It is no wonder either that those who approach the world with the greatest sense of wonder and the most sensitivity to the mysteries of nature are scientists and mystics, frequently in the same person. In China this line of development is even more clear, and historically it has been the Taoist tradition which largely has been responsible for the development of Chinese medicine, astronomy, chemistry and botany. Other traditions, such as Confucianism, with its obsessive concern for right-action, duty, and the following of man-made conventions, have understandably been unproductive in these areas. "Scientific" interests and methods quite naturally grew out of Taoist concerns. The interest in immortality, for example, led to the growth of Chinese medicine, as well as exhaustive compilations of information on plants, herbs, medicines, and their uses. The Chinese *Pen Ts'ao, The Great Pharmacopoeia,* an exhaustive work in fifty-two volumes, is part of the Taoist canon. Disciplines like Tai Chi have their origins in this strain of Taoism with its interest in

166

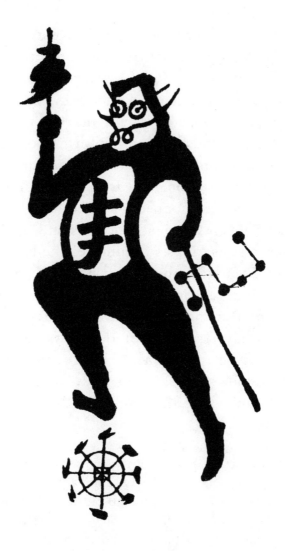

Popular Taoism has a rich tradition of talismans which were seen as being inhabited by spirits. The talismans acted as mediums between this world and the world of the spirits. This example is of the Messenger of the Nine Heavens who has the power to cure disease. (From the *Tao-tsang*).

167

immortality, prolonging life, and promoting good health.

All of this is not to say that Taoism doesn't have its share of wild speculation, fuzzy-headedness, and popularized magic. Even Chuang Tzu, writing in the fourth century B.C. was concerned with making a distinction between the genuine and the uninformed or corrupt. Some scholars have taken these critical remarks — combined with their own personal needs to see Lao Tzu and Chuang Tzu as "pure" philosophers — and attempted to show that mystical Taoism was just a debasement of their thought. This approach seriously diminishes the breadth of Taoist thought. Even the abstract concepts had a reality for them, and were conceived of as being more than just metaphors. Chuang Tzu writes of the Tao as a real place. "I myself have traversed it this way and that; yet still know only where it begins. I have roamed at will through its stupendous spaces. I know how to get to them, but I do not know where they end." Of the Yin and the Yang he writes:

> I saw Yin the Female Energy, in its motionless grandeur; I saw Yang, the Male Energy rampant in its fiery vigour. The motionless grandeur came up out of the earth; the fiery vigour burst out from heaven. The two penetrated one another, were inextricably blended and from their union the things of the world were born.

In the third and fourth centuries B.C. there were many schools dealing with both the spiritual and physical aspects of meditation. One school of thought, which Arthur Waley calls the "School of Chi", held that weakness in man, both moral and physical, came from a shrinking of his vital energies, or life-spirit, or "chi". The best of mankind were those whose whole bodies were pervaded with "chi". With sufficient "chi" everything was possible, and the secret lay in accumulating and storing this "chi" in the body.

> Never till that pool [of chi] runs dry shall the Four Limbs fail:
> Nor till the well is exhausted shall the traffic of the
>   Nine Apertures cease.
> Thereby shall you be enabled to explore Heaven and Earth,
> Reach the Four Oceans that bound the world;
> Within, have no thoughts that perplex,
> Without, suffer no evil or calamity.
> Inside, the mind shall be whole;
> Whole too the bodily frame.

From *The Way and Its Power*, Arthur Waley

Here is one of the sources of Tai Chi, an art specifically designed to cultivate this "chi". The benefits derived include not only mental and physical integrity, but the power to explore the whole world, and to be free of human suffering.

Many of these ideas had a common currency in the Taoist thought of the third and fourth centuries B.C. Some men however, not content with improved health and longevity, insisted that the ultimate goal should be immor-

169

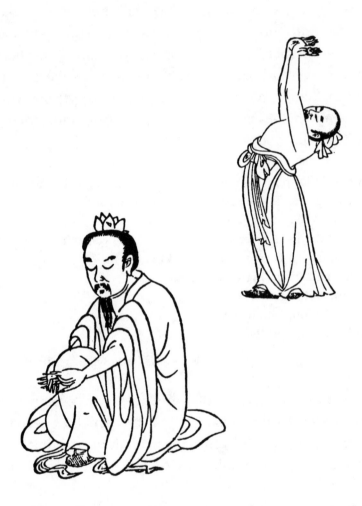

A concentration exercise for the fourth month and a stretching exercise for the fifth month. To be practiced daily between the hours of one and three A.M.

170

tality. A number of manuals survive that describe in great detail the requisite techniques. There is even a tract written by a living Taoist scholar, Lu K'uan Yu, which exhaustively describes this process. In essence the technique involves transforming the semen by means of the breath and mind to create a chemical in the body which promotes health, and results ultimately in the creation of a spirit body which survives the physical body. A kind of do-it-yourself internal alchemy.

Alchemy has always had two faces, one concerned with finding the *prima materia*, the original substance, in the natural world, and using this discovery to transmute metals and other physical substances, e.g. to change lead into gold. The other face of alchemy turned inward and hoped to find this same *elixir of life* within, using psychic or spiritual techniques. In this instance the primary goal was immortality, and only secondarily included the ability to transform material substances. The Buddhist tradition is filled with stories of the miraculous accomplishments of those who have come to this knowledge, and the tradition is still very much alive. The exterior alchemical tradition, to a large degree, was incorporated into modern science in the West, and the quest continues among nuclear physicists to find the alchemists *prima materia*.

In Taoist meditation, and in Tai Chi, the alchemical process begins at the base of the spine. The "chi" is tapped at the sacrum and then proceeds up the spine. When

171

you watch a Tai Chi master move you can see the force rippling up the spine from the bottom to the top. This energy is stored in a spot just below the navel, called the "tan-tien". This point is roughly equivalent to a Yogic "chakra", appears in Sufi thought, and is described in Castaneda's *The Teachings of Don Juan: A Yaqui Way of Knowledge.*

In Tai Chi the energy travels from the sacrum to the ends of the fingers, circles back to the body, and then moves down to the "tan-tien". In Taoist meditation this "chi" is circulated internally. *The Secret of the Golden Flower* describes this process. "The way leads from the sacrum upward in a backward manner to the summit of the Creative; then it sinks through two stories in a downward-flowing way in the solar plexus and warms it. Therefore it is said: Wandering in Heaven one eats the spirit-power of the receptive. Because the true power goes back into the empty place in time, power and form become right and full, body and heart glad and cheerful."

One of the secrets of Tai Chi, as well as alchemy, lies in the subtle relationship of the mind to the body. The two are thought to act as one. *The Secret of the Golden Flower* talks about this relationship in some detail. "Action in non-action prevents man from sinking into numbing emptiness and dead nothingness. When the Heavenly Heart [mind] still preserves calm movement before the right time it is a fault of softness. When the Heavenly Heart has already moved, the movement that follows afterwards, corresponding with it, is a fault of rigidity." The ideal quality of the movements in Tai Chi lies somewhere between complete relaxation and tension, somewhere between rigidness and flaccidness. What gives the movement life is this precise coordination of the mind — or the Heavenly Heart — and the body.

For all of this deliberateness, the other half of the secret lies in being able to release, to uncouple, to do nothing to our bodies. Our bodies know how to work very well without our interference. In the same way that we wouldn't dream of consciously assuming control of the functioning of the liver, or the generation of brain cells — knowing that these organs and cells have complete instructions on how to function that are far too complicated for our conscious minds to follow — so we should learn to give in, to stop interfering with the external workings of our bodies, and to let them work the way they were meant to. In *Journey to Ixtlan* Don Juan tells Carlos just this: "I've told you that the secret of a strong body is not in what you do to it but in what you don't do."

In both Tai Chi and meditation sensitivity to the flow of energy is essential for development, and this sensitivity is the product of mental concentration. The concentration is of a specific sort though, not what we associate with furrowed brows, gritted teeth, and perplexed expressions. Rather it is a non-specific attentiveness. Most of the attention naturally should be on performing the Tai Chi movements, but a good deal of the time, for most people, there will also be a part of the mind that is worried about doing the form better, that is going over a disturbing conversation from several hours before, that is annoyed about noise from the street. Rather than trying to force these thoughts out of the mind it is enough just to be aware of what the thoughts are, to note them, but not to dwell on them. It is a form of violence — and one that requires considerable energy — to be constantly editing these thoughts, fighting with ourselves to repress them, getting angry with ourselves for our particularly mean or petty ones. But the Tai Chi form itself which follows the natural rhythms of our own breathing, soothes the mind as the body moves, and even for beginning students there will be times when the inner struggles cease. The breathing can in the course of doing Tai Chi, become so quietly internalized that it almost seems to stop. In Taoist meditation this state is deliberately sought.

> One should not be able to hear with the ear the outgoing and intaking of the breath. What one hears is that it has no tone. As soon as it has tone, the breathing is rough and superficial and does not penetrate into what is fine. Then the heart must be made quite light and insignificant. The more it is relaxed, the less important it becomes; the less important, the quieter. All at once it becomes so quiet that it stops.
>
> *The Secret of the Golden Flower*

174

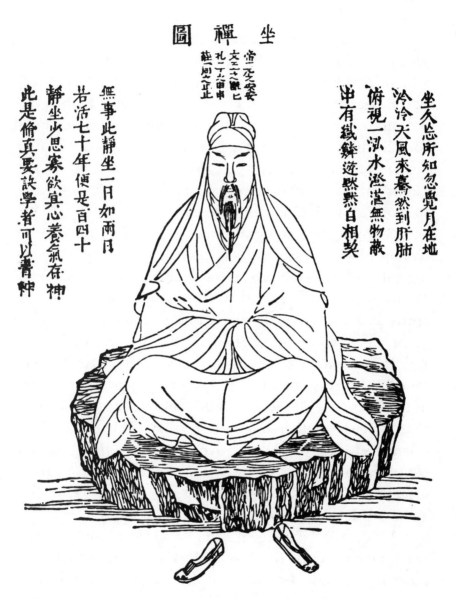

坐
禪
圖

坐久忽所知忽覺月在地
冷冷天風來颯然到肝肺
俯視一泓水澄澄無物瑕
中有纖鱗遊黙黙自相笑

無事此靜坐一日如兩日
若活七十年便是百四十
靜坐少思寮欲寡心養氣存神
此是偷真要訣學者可以菁神

當二至之安
文王之六六二盥已
孔一大田申
莊一同入止此

The first stage of meditation, the accumulation of light.
T'ai I Chin Hua Tsung Chih.

175

Tai Chi Ch'uan

This quietness is a reflection of an inner stillness, and it is this inner stillness that is at the heart of all spiritual techniques. Described in a slightly different way, bringing an end to our internal conversations is the foundation for a greater awareness, and the real starting point for all kinds of mystical and magical practices. In Don Juan's words, "the crux of sorcery is the internal dialogue; that is the key to everything. When a warrior learns to stop it, everything becomes possible."

Stopping this internal dialogue, in turn, results in a feeling of lightness which is both physical and psychological, and with it comes a sense of joy. In *The Secret of the Golden Flower* we read: "If when there is quiet, the spirit has continuously and uninterruptedly a sense of great gaiety as if intoxicated or freshly bathed, it is a sign that the light principle in the whole body is harmonious." With this comes a dissipation of our normal fears and anxieties. "The whole body feels strong and firm so that it fears neither storm nor frost. Things by which other men are displeased, when I meet them, cannot cloud the brightness of the Seed of the Spirit." There is a feeling of relief, of reconciliation, and the sense that some burden has been removed.

In the Taoist texts this joy and sense of lightness is thought to be the result of a chemical change that takes place in the body. Our altered physical and mental states when meditating or doing Tai Chi clearly must have a chemical component. The obvious question is whether

176

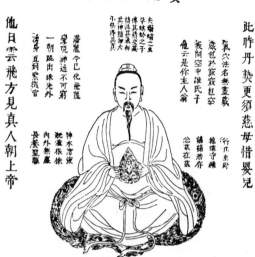

要兒現形圖

他日雲飛方見真人朝上帝

落寞今已化飛龍
瑩現神通不可窮
一朝跳出珠光外
渾身且到紫微宮

夫嬰兒之生
孕蛻於之中
傳其神矣乎
精氣其無不
其神隨出大
小然得其大

氣穴法名無盡藏
溫包於竅寂紅空
我間空中誰氏子
他云是你主人翁

行住坐臥
龍蟠守雌
綿綿若存
念茲在茲

神水溶溶
沉潛根炁
內外無塵
長養聖胎

此時丹熟更須慈母惜嬰兒

The beginnings of the new being at the power center.
T'ai I Chin Hua Tsung Chih.

The point at which the spirit-body separates from the physical body
and begins a separate existence.

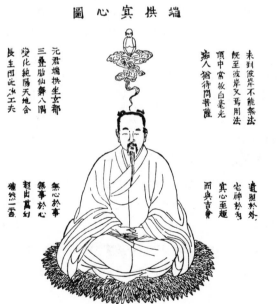

端拱冥心圖

長生問此火工夫
煅化純陽天地合
三疊胎仙舞八隅
元君端拱坐玄都

確然一畨
超出萬幻
無事於心
無心於事

未到彼岸不能無法
既至彼岸又焉用法
頂中常放白毫光
冥心至趣

癡人猶待問菩薩

遺照於外
宅神於內
而與吉會

177

this body alchemy is not part of the same process that psychologists and psychiatrists are now studying and experimenting with using chemicals and drugs. It will not surprise us if at some point the two traditions arrive at roughly the same conclusions.

We frequently forget that thought has a physical aspect, that the messages the brain sends are as real as letters we send in the mail. The mental part of Tai Chi has a decidedly physical character, and is effective to the degree these mental messages dominate our mental processes at any given moment. This is another way of saying that if our minds are clear and focussed on one image, that image, or message, has more impact than if we have a number of things floating through our heads at the same time. In Chögyam Trungpa's book *Meditation in Action* there is a good description of our ordinary mental process: "One thought comes and almost before we finish that another one comes in and overlaps it and then another. So we never allow any gap which would permit us to be free and really digest things." When we can get out of this pattern there is a sense of relief — frequently a sense of great weariness as though we are finally able to rest our minds after years and years of incessant use. We create the space in which to look at the world and ourselves free of the burden of distraction. Meditation is "The teaching of letting the mind be in a very open way, of feeling the flow of energy without trying to subdue it and without letting it get out of control, of going with the energy pattern of mind. . . . Such practice is necessary generally because our thinking pattern, our conceptualized way of conducting our life in the world is either too manipulative, imposing itself upon the world, or else runs completely wild and uncontrolled. Therefore, our meditation practice must begin with ego's outermost layer, the discursive thoughts which continually run through our minds, our mental gossip." (*Cutting Through Spiritual Materialism* by Chögyam Trungpa.)

In Tai Chi this subtle balance between holding on too tightly and letting go completely is learned both in the mind and in the body. The carry-over of Tai Chi into our everyday lives is made smoother because we are in a state half-way between a still and internal meditative state and a more external, active state. The description of Tai Chi Ch'uan as meditation in motion is an apt one.

Ultimately though we are not talking about changes in our bodies and minds as a result of meditation or Tai Chi. Our concern is with what happens to us as whole people. "The key is this", writes Jung, "We must be able to let things happen in the psyche. For us this becomes a real art of which few people know anything. Consciousness is forever interfering, helping, correcting, negating, never leaving the simple growth of the psyche in peace."

But just how "simple" is this process of growth in the psyche? It is easy enough to talk about just letting things happen, but not so easy when we grasp the extent to which our education, training and experience has taught us to *make* things happen; to plan, to acquire information, to make and keep as much money as possible, to preserve experience. One of the things that is so strategic about Tai Chi in this struggle is that it doesn't approach these questions on their own terms. It isn't a process of trying to reason with the mind, or of convincing us that it is in our interests to be this way and not that way. Tai Chi goes directly to the body. And through a process that is endlessly repetitive, the body learns. "When one does something with people", Don Juan tells Carlos, "the concern should be only with presenting the case to their bodies. That's what I've been doing with you so far, letting your body know. Who cares whether or not you understand." Our bodies fortunately are not capable of guile or evasion like our minds. Our bodies have much to teach us.

In the course of practicing Tai Chi there are major alterations in our familiar perceptions of the world. We fall into the changes so effortlessly that at times we aren't even aware that anything is different. Our sense of time is slowed down so that we can feel every instant of time, every inch of movement. It is like moving in a dream, or like movement shown in slow motion on film. There is a common experience in Tai Chi of seemingly falling through a hole in time. Awareness of the passage of time completely stops, and only when you catch yourself, after five or ten minutes, or five or ten seconds, is there the

180

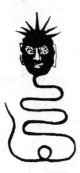

Taoist talisman from the *Tao-tsang*. This talisman is of the Supreme Ruler of the South Pole who has the powers to order the other spirits.

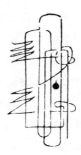

Taoist talisman, this one is of the Ruler of the South who assists the process of becoming an immortal. *(Tao-tsang)*.

Taoist talisman from the *Tao-tsang* requesting aid from the Supreme Jade Sovereign.

realization that for that period of time the world *stopped*. During that period the movements have continued, but without the aid of the conscious part of our minds which we assume to be essential for precise physical activity.

Our perception of space is also altered. This happens on two levels. As the air thickens around our bodies while we do Tai Chi, we have a sense of moving through this heavier medium. To do this our bodies get weightier, and there is a feeling of actually expanding in space. There is also a much more subtle expansion of our awareness outside the narrow confines of what is immediately around us. There is a sense of our "chi" actually flowing out from us into the larger space in which we move. Paradoxically this results in a much clearer sense of where we are, and where our center is. Centered, still, our breathing almost inaudible, there comes a marked improvement in our hearing, as though someone suddenly unplugged our ears.

Mentally, somewhere between a state of artificial excitement and a state of inflexible discipline, between the emotions and the will, lies the ideal state of mind for practicing Tai Chi — a state of simple awareness. This awareness is an emptiness that exists between our accumulation of bodily and mental memorabilia, and our future expectations of the something better that is in store for us. The personification of this quality of awareness is the warrior. It is remarkable how often and in what disparate traditions this image appears, not only in Tai Chi, which after all has a martial side, but in meditational tracts and yogic writings. "A great warrior", as one meditational text puts it "has no opinions, he is simply aware". To be a warrior is to be self-possessed, centered, acutely aware, and empty. It is a very particular state of mind, one which focusses on the moment, free of doubts and idle speculations. "In a world where death is the hunter, my friend, there is not time for regrets or doubts. There is only time for decisions."

A NOTE ON SOURCES

The references in this chapter come from a fairly motley collection of sources which reflect wanderings in this literature over the past decade, as well as some systematic reading on meditation and Tai Chi. The collection of books written by Carlos Castaneda and published by Simon and Schuster have been influential. Whether or not Don Juan is a real character — which has been questioned — seems incidental to the content of the books. Carlos on the other hand is a perfectly believable sorcerer's apprentice, and a comic foil to the "impeccable" Don Juan. Carlos is fat, out of shape, pedantic, has a troubled relationship with his parents, is on the one hand completely gullible and on the other a thoroughgoing skeptic, and in the clinch, when confronted with the mysteries of the universe, reaches for his notebook to write about the experiences. The four books are: *Tales of Power, Journey to Ixtlan, A Separate Reality,* and *The Teachings of Don Juan: A Yaqui Way of Knowledge.* On Taoist meditation and alchemy I have relied heavily on *The Secret of the Golden Flower: A Chinese Book of Life,* translated by Richard Wilhelm, with a commentary by C. G. Jung, Causeway Books, New York, 1975. The same characters who brought you the *I Ching.* This is a difficult, but rich text. Also *Taoist Yoga: Alchemy and Immortality,* by Lu K'uan Yu, Samuel Weiser, New York, 1973. A very complex, though apparently complete how-to-do-it book on becoming an immortal. "The book is reverently dedicated to my godfather, the Deity Pe Ti, ruler of the Northern Heaven, who has helpfully guided me in my translation of Taoist Scriptures herein presented." *Buddhist Meditation,* Edward Conze, Harper and Row, New York, 1969 is quite different in style from the Taoist texts, but equally rich. A nice book of first hand experiences with Taoist recluses and mystics is *The Secret and Sublime: Taoist Mysteries and Magic* by John Blofeld, E. P. Dutton, New York, 1973. Where Blofeld's book on the I Ching is a little stuffy, this one is light, entertaining, and very personable. There is a new book on *Tao Magic: The Chinese Art of the Occult* by Laszlo Legeza, Pantheon Books, New York, 1975. This text has beautiful illustrations and an informative text.

Chögyam Trungpa is the eleventh incarnation of the Trungpa Tulku and was raised from childhood to be the supreme abbot of the Surmang monasteries in eastern Tibet. Forced to leave Tibet he has taken up residence in this country and written a number of excellent books; among them *Meditation in Action* and *Cutting Through Spiritual Materialism* both published by Shambhala Publications, Berkeley, California.

A very different sort of book is *Autobiography of a Yogi* by Paramahansa Yogananda, Self-Realization Fellowship, Los Angeles, 1973 — fascinating, mind boggling, at times a not altogether believable book.

Finally, a very informative book, *Foundations of Tibetan Mysticism: According to the Esoteric Teachings of the Great Mantra Om Padme Hun* by Lama Anagarika Govinda, Rider & Co., London, 1960.

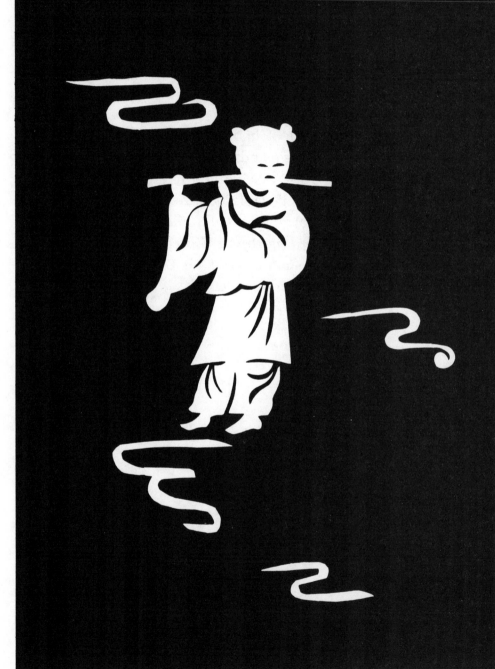

Tai Chi and Dance:
The Techniques of Power

> *In America many people live in their bodies like in abandoned houses, haunted with memories of when they were occupied.*
>
> Joseph Chaiken

We must begin by accepting that the body exists in a physical universe, and is subject to the laws of that universe. The central area of the human body is its base of power. The body is strongest and most stable when it acknowledges gravity and can manipulate the play of its weight against the earth. But if you look around downtown one day you will see that the human world is filled with distorted and unnatural shapes. Business men and others with sedentary jobs are afflicted by a kind of top-heaviness — the chests are much too large for the hips and legs. Women, with a lower center of gravity and more of their mass in the hips, find it more natural to "sink the weight", in accordance with the principles of Tai Chi. But all too often this natural female shape is grossly exaggerated by bad eating habits and little exercise. The hips spread out and immobilize the body.

Our current problems are the result of a long process of natural history. As a two-legged creature came into being, the hands were freed from the need to help support and locomote. As the hands took over the job of holding and carrying from the mouth, the head was freed. And here we are, talking and thinking, lawyers, doctors, and Indian Chiefs. But now we are finally becoming conscious of the destruction left behind in the wake of our remarkable advances. We are paying a high price because we have severed ourselves from our visceral connection to the universe, in the name of intelligence and the "higher" functions of mind.

Western medicine, which has largely to do with the diagnosis of disease and severe malfunction, knows precious little about exercise and other preventative systems. It is neither useless nor unintelligent, only incomplete. There are ways, and ways, of knowing. Tai Chi fills a serious gap, keeping the body strong so that it can heal itself from day to day. It is used therapeutically, here and in China, for heart and lung problems. Even someone who is quite weak can do some version of the exercise, however limited, and still benefit.

The question for many people is, what kind of exercise should I do, and how much of it do I have to do in order to stay fit? On the most basic level the question of fitness has to do with the body's ability to combine oxygen with food stored in the body to produce energy. While the body can store food, it cannot store oxygen, so our heart and lungs and circulatory system are constantly working to keep things going. Being fit means that the body has efficient systems for doing this.

Most of us are capable of meeting the requirements of our bodies in our daily lives, but what happens in situations where our bodies require more energy: when we are sick, when we can't get enough rest, when we are under great stress? Then we need reserves, reserves which can only be produced by exercising on a regular basis.

Exercise can build a stronger and more efficient heart which pumps more blood with each stroke. You can increase the capacity of the circulatory system by actually increasing the number of blood vessels and the volume of blood in the body. Lower blood pressure results from a more conditioned circulatory system. The lungs increase their ability to bring in oxygen and to process it, so that the capacity of the lungs to consume oxygen increases.

Proper exercise requires, for a period of time, increasing the heart rate and the consumption of oxygen, while neither straining the heart nor robbing the body of the oxygen which it needs at any moment. (Sprinting, for example, while it conditions the leg muscles, creates

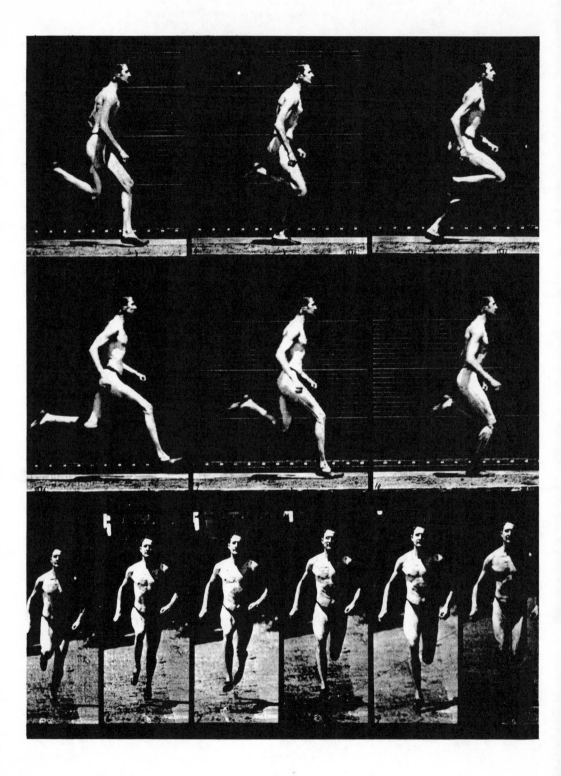

an oxygen deficit.) Healthful exercise is moderate and continuous over a fairly long period of time. Because it satisfies all of these conditions, Tai Chi is an ideal exercise.

ALIGNMENT — THE BODY AT REST

One of the basic lessons of Tai Chi is alignment, or what we used to call posture. A body in alignment balances the various weights as they accumulate downward and are transferred through the feet to the ground. Like everything else in the world we are subject to the downward force of gravity, and our feet are rather a narrow base to support the mass of the body with its heavy bones and viscera. The muscles work through alternating rhythms of rest and activity, although a healthy body will always maintain muscle tone — a minimal state of contraction and elasticity. If the bony weights of the body do not hang in balance, muscle must be used to support and compensate for the structural strain — a condition which leads to constant fatigue. Instead of being ready for movement, the muscles are tired and need rest. This kind of muscular fatigue can even persist through sleep. When people first start Tai Chi, their bodies usually show overwhelming tension — a sad legacy of our ignorance about natural alignment. It is of crucial importance that the bones which support the viscera be in proper alignment so that energy is not continually dissipated by unnecessary muscular strain.

If the skeleton is balanced it will hang downward — no parts should be held away from the center. Most of us, unfortunately, do not grow into our bodies in accordance with these natural structural principles. You could find the origin of your own postural peculiarities if you could remember how you felt about yourself and your body as a child or pre-adolescent, and what you were taught about posture by well-meaning but ill informed teachers and parents. Too tall? Too short? Too flat-chested or too bosomy? Frightened, shrinking? Those habits dig in early and deep, until we lose completely any dependable sense of what "feels" natural and comfortable.

The most cursory study of anatomy and kinesthesiology will demonstrate the incredible interdependence of the systems of the human body. Nothing happens to any part of it without reverberating deeply through the entire organism.

If the bones are not balanced, muscles are used to compensate. But breathing also is a muscular activity and suffers when the necessary muscles cannot be used fully because they are straining to make up for structural imbalance. In turn, when you cannot breathe deeply the muscles cannot relax because they do not receive sufficient oxygen. And the tension in the muscles constricts the blood vessels so the capacity of the circulatory system is seriously diminished. And on it goes.

While doing Tai Chi the knees and ankles are always bent, and the chest is slightly pulled back, or softened, so that the weight is lined up over the heels. The joints are relaxed, and the body "hangs" from the crown of the head as if suspended from above. This posture is the easiest one in which to sense the correct alignment of the bones and to be conscious of balance through the joints. Modern Dance and ballet are based on similar principles of alignment — of course the human body is still the human body. But the dancer stands on straightened legs, and balances the weight over the balls of the feet preparing to rise up on a stretched arch, and to jump. In this position it is much trickier to sense good skeletal alignment.

To demonstrate this to yourself, stand in front of a mirror with your knees bent so you are reflected in profile. Bend your knees comfortably and experiment with your pelvic area, watching your ass. You will find that you can either tuck it underneath you, or push it out behind you, or let it hang directly downward beneath you. In this last position your spine takes its longest and most released curve, properly supported by the wall of abdominal muscles in front. When you have found that place, very slowly stretch your legs. Keep your eyes on the area of the lower spine — it is easy, as you stretch the knees, to let the pelvis tip up and protrude in the back, shortening the curve of the spine and throwing the body out of alignment.

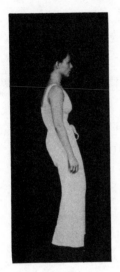
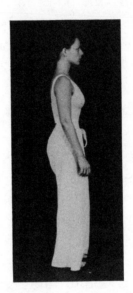
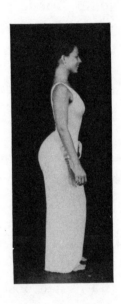

Alignment — The Body at Rest

With the knees slightly bent we can easily feel three main postural
possibilities. The pelvis can be tucked under, relaxed straight downwards, or tilted up and out in the back. This last possibility is the
dangerous one. We hear often of a painful and mysterious lower back
ailment, apparently undiagnosable. This is no mystery, but the result
of a life-time's accumulation of structural strain. The abdominal muscles are not used properly to support the viscera and the back-bone
bears a burden for which it is not prepared.

194

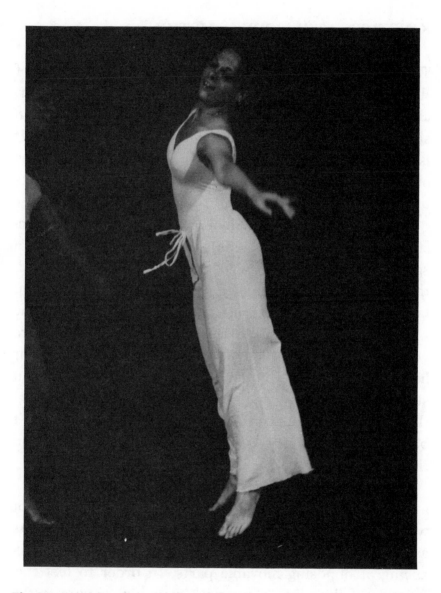

The Western dancer must always be prepared to rise up on the balls of the feet or on the toes, and to jump.

Tai Chi Ch'uan

KINETICS — THE BODY IN MOTION

The Tai Chi movements are based on an acceptance of the human body and the ways in which it moves naturally. The body is dynamic, in constant motion; even in sleep it is constantly re-adjusting a delicate balance. It is easier in fact to move than it is to stand still, as everyone discovers posing for photographs or waiting for pants to be shortened.

One of the bases for human locomotion is the principle of functional opposition. The body walks with a spiral action. When you walk and one leg steps forward, the arm opposite to that leg swings forward. When you take the next step the arms reverse, swinging from the shoulders. Nobody has to think about this; if you are walking along without anything to carry in your arms or hands this swinging motion is natural and easy. If you stop and try to take one step at a time, thinking about the "principle of opposition", as likely as not you won't be able to do it. The conscious mind is often far behind the body.

Opposition originates in the center of the body with a twisting of the spine. It is the most efficient way of walking (or running or whatever) since it keeps all parts as close to the center as possible. It is a dynamic balancing of opposing movable parts. In order to feel this twisting of the spine, stand with your hips square to the front of the room and rotate your torso first to one side and then to the other, initiating the movement from the waist and not from the shoulders. You can't move very far, but you can feel the spine twist — the action is similar to wringing out a wet cloth, spiralling the top against the bottom.

The limbs are connected to the central body by rotary joints. Both hips and shoulders are a kind of ball and socket. I was surprised to learn that these joints are only very loosely bound by connective tissue and are held together mostly by suction. It is simple mechanics that the limbs (especially the arms which have no part in supporting weight) relate to the central body as spokes to the hub of a wheel, swinging around from the joint. When Tai Chi is done properly, no matter what form or style is practiced, the arms never move in isolation from the rest of the body. The principle is that all movement begins in the center and returns to the center. The waist swings and the arms circle effortlessly in their joints, with no strain or muscular force. The impetus of movement lies in the joint rather than in the outstretched arm. This is an efficient principle — known and practiced by all competent golfers, tennis players, etc. The strength and mass of the body is in its center, so it makes sense to begin and control motion at the waist.

Consider this illustration. Hold one end of a long belt in one hand. Imagine that end to be the center of a circle, with a radius equal to the length of the belt. If you try to describe the periphery of the circle by using your

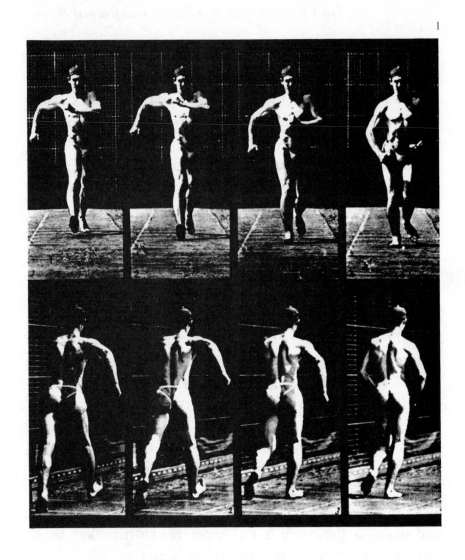

MAN WALKING AT HALF-STRIDE (.069 second)
Eadweard Muybridge (Dover)

The principle of functional opposition—the body walks, runs, throws, with a spiral action.

198

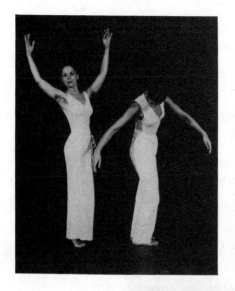
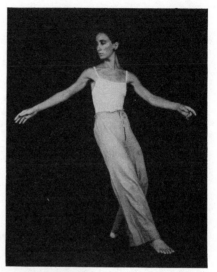

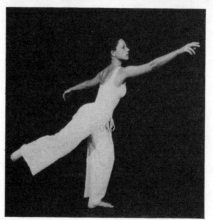

The dancer rotates the torso against the hips or the standing leg. Tai Chi is based on the same principle of opposition — the solid, supporting leg transmits its strength through the waist and sacrum diagonally to the opposite hand and arm.

199

other hand to move the free end of the belt, your efforts will be slow and awkward. However, if you leave one end to swing free, and merely flip the wrist of the hand holding the "center" end, the belt will swing around and around, smoothly and with great speed.

Beginning at the center; returning to the center. Tai Chi is basically a conservative philosophy of motion. Conservative as in conservation, not as in Ronald Reagan. One of the priorities is simply to endure — energy flows in circles, always returning, never exhausted. This is a kind of thinking that we are beginning to understand as we foresee that in the near future we may have exhausted the world's once "inexhaustible" energy reserves. Tai Chi is also recycling of energy — and it demonstrates that for each of us our bodies can be a microcosm of the whole physical universe.

*　　*　　*

CHI — THE SOURCE OF POWER

"Chi", a Chinese word, is an elusive term. It is not readily translatable into English but means something like intrinsic energy, inner strength, breath energy, etc. It is said to be stored in the center of the body — in a spot about two inches below the navel. At first glance the more skeptical Western mind may dismiss "chi" as some kind of hocus-pocus, but it is familiar to everyone. We have all "seen" chi in action. When first you look at a group of moving dancers, your eye wanders, not focusing on anyone in particular. Suddenly some motion calls your eye — that dancer has chi. When you watch a skilled athlete perform an act you know to be very difficult, requiring great strength, and it is done with such ease and completion that it seems to happen by itself — that athlete has chi. I see chi often out of the corner of my eye, with my most peripheral vision. In a roomful of students practicing, my eye is caught and pulled by a palpable wave of energy, when someone gets a movement just right. It is easier to describe than to define, this experience of finding the "flow" in any motion so that energy is released without any abrupt force or strain. It is a physical discovery — there is a limit to how much you can teach this kind of thing through verbal explanation. The body learns through repetition; it does not always require the intervention of the conscious mind. Sometimes you discover your chi in moments of great stress or panic when you perform, without thinking, an otherwise "impossible" feat of strength.

It is a sorry fact that most of us in our everyday lives are able to mobilize only a tiny fraction of our potential energy. We are drained by our tension and fatigue, limited by the pressures of our lives and our physical ignorance. The inner strength of chi is not a magic trick. Enormous energy is available to the body that knows how to relax, that is well-balanced and grounded and initiates motion from the center, always returning to the center. Tai Chi is practiced in slow motion, enabling you to become conscious of the circulation of the chi, and to follow the pathways of your own energy. The form is an empty shell, filled with inner vitality. In giving form to energy, the spirit is made physical. Practicing slowly, over and over, the body unlearns the inefficient tension of years and re-discovers a more natural and easy strength.

The basic principles of Tai Chi are the same as those of any effective and efficient physical exercise, whether it be for sport or art. Any athlete or dancer who has carefully refined a potential for motion demonstrates in his or her technique the knowledge, conscious or not, of the circular nature of motion. The rest of us often enough agree in recogniziing it, although we call it by many different names. Animals and small babies are blessed with the same knowledge, in the course of things, without practice or study.

Effort is not the same thing as stress. You know you have mastered something when it begins to come easily. If energy is circulating, always returning, always accumulating, then exercise is revitalizing, not draining. Some very strenuous activities leave one feeling high, exhilarated. But a short time later, exhaustion sets in. The body has borrowed on its energy reserves. Hysterical scenes and frantic concentrated activity also produce this feeling of "speediness", followed by an unpleasant crash. Tai

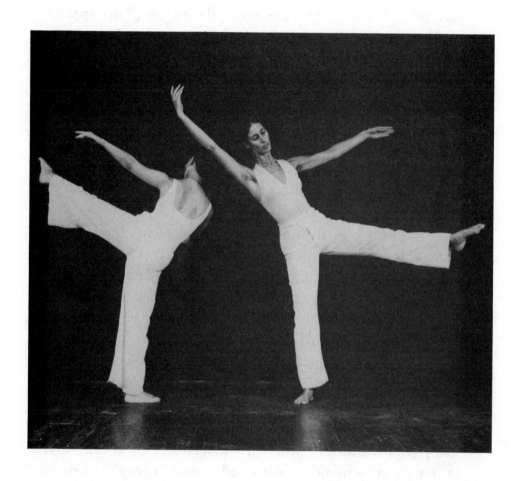

In dance as well as in Tai Chi the performer cultivates the skill of balance on one leg. The "empty" leg is freed to extend and rotate at the hip socket.

Chi is always replenishing the body's reserves — taking in a little more than is extended outward.

Among other things dancing is about flight — the liberation from weight, and from the earth. (This applies to modern Western dancing and is not true of dance in many other cultures.) This is achieved, paradoxically, by a very refined manipulation of weight itself. The dancer flies through the air not because the body is weightless, but because weight is transcended through the skillful use of it. In dancing many natural possibilities of the human body are refined and exaggerated. The dancer learns by hard and tedious practice how to use the reality of the body — the small internal muscles, the delicate counter-pulls — in an endless effort to realize the "ideal" form. This "ideal" comes mostly from the curious and out-dated aesthetic of classical ballet. The body should be long and lean, incredibly "turned out" in the hip joints and stretched through the back. Women must not be too tall; men must not be too short. The "ideal" female dancer ought to look as much as possible like a fourteen-year-old boy. Most dancers have been told at some point that they just do not have the "right" body. Often dancers with bodies that are naturally plump and fleshy quite literally starve themselves. The energy loss is temporarily made up with coffee and "speed". In some sense, dancing is an attempt to train the body to come closer and closer to this ideal standard.

Anyone can rotate the legs in the hip socket to some

204

extent; anyone can learn to attenuate the muscles of the arms and legs. But there always exist the limitations of natural and acquired disparities of body awareness, muscle tone, bone structure, etc. Tai Chi is a form which allows each body the discovery of itself. Tai Chi uses the laws of biology and physics to teach the body to grow, and to change, and to recharge itself as long as there is life. In this sense there is no final limitation. When an athlete trains to run the mile, for example, at some point he will reach his limit, his best speed. But Tai Chi grows always deeper.

How does it happen that athletes and dancers, who presumably are trained to use their bodies in accordance with "natural" principles, are so prone to injury? Particular sports often emphasize or over-use one part of the body. Dancers suffer injuries through over-stretching. The standard is the ideal. In working to rotate the hips and stretch the muscles, further and further and further, some bodies stretch beyond their strength, losing a kind of natural protection. Injury results from over-use or from specialization at the cost of the integrity of the whole — tennis elbow, football knees, etc. The competitive emphasis on speed and victory above all else can change a healthy exercise, over a period of time, into punishment.

Ballet companies must constantly change their programs because of injury. In fact, in the world of sports and in the world of dance, the activity as an end in itself

205

is valued far and above the health and well-being of the performers. The general unwritten ethos glorifies persistence in spite of injury, and at the cost of even greater injury. "The show must go on" etc., etc. Anyone involved in the theatre or professional sports can tell a few ghastly stories about dancing with third degree burns or playing hockey with wired jaws. Sometimes the stress creates a secondary injury, but all the stories are told with great relish.

No one who has experienced the glorious exhilaration of dancing, as performer, audience, or student, would want to take away any of its incredible sense of flight and freedom. But underlying the glory is an implicit hierarchy of values. A price is paid, and much is lost along the way.

Of course there is no point in setting up a contest between Tai Chi and dancing, arguing which is more natural, or which more beautiful. The practice of Tai Chi has much to teach any student of dance. There are the obvious things — balance, centeredness, and continuity of motion. The slowness of the motion of Tai Chi, moving as if under water, heightens the body's consciousness of space. The air around the body takes on a viscous quality. Space, the dancer's medium, becomes real and substantial.

From the endless alternating rhythms of Tai Chi the dancer learns contrast and dynamic. To "play" Tai Chi is to experience the flow of energy from within. The alternating forces of the universe make themselves mani-

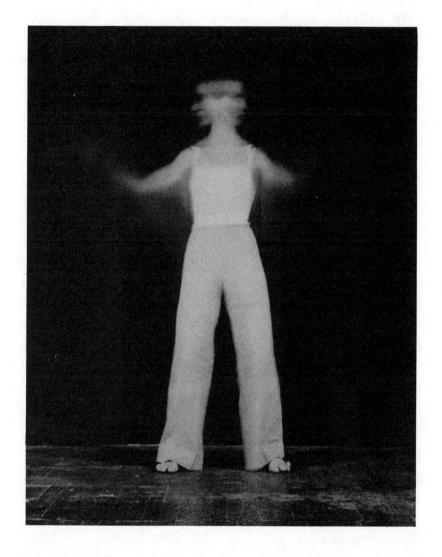

The limbs relate to the central body as spokes to the hub of a wheel.

fest in each body that lives and breathes. Essentially (and this is even true, in a basic sense, for the traditional narrative ballet) dancing too is just this:

> . . . a play of Powers made visible . . . The first recognition of them (the Powers that surround humanity) is through the feeling of personal power and will in the human body and their first representation is through a bodily activity which abstracts the sense of power from the practical experience in which that sense is usually an obscure factor. This activity is known as dancing.
>
> Langer

Each discipline has something to teach the other; neither is a substitute for the other. I am even reluctant to make the obvious remark — that not everyone can dance, while everyone, old *or* young, well or ill, can do Tai Chi. Not everyone has the drive, the talent, or the desire to become a performing dancer. But anyone *can* dance. There is nothing quite like the feeling of leaping or running across a big open space to the beat of the drum. And although it is not in everyone to become a concert dancer, any serious student can learn from dancing its lesson of vulnerability and patience. Again and again I am struck as I watch beginning adult dance classes by the courage it takes to try — to be willing to stumble and fall like an awkward child, to be willing to expose yourself to failure, publicly, over and over again. Physical disciplines demand to be learned from the "inside out", and the first step is always to unlearn. No matter how much you would like to be able to lift your leg up to your ear, you must *begin* with the most minimal extension, carefully aligning the center of the body, unlearning old habits of tension and strain. In order to move forward you must begin from where *you* are. Learning Tai Chi, shifting the weight slowly from one leg to another, there is no way to pretend you are balanced if you are not. The body does not lie. You begin here.

"Ideal" form and natural limitations create a hierarchy of performers, at its worst in the "star" system of classical ballet. There is also always the division between those who dance and those who watch. You *can* watch Tai Chi but it does not depend upon any other presence. It is a meditative solitary activity. Like meditation, you practice in order to be able to extend the meditative consciousness until it is with you every minute, in everything you do. You don't rest after Tai Chi, or catch your breath, or slump with relief. It stretches through all the hours of your days.

Modern dancing makes a distinction between technique and the end — the work — which technique serves. The study of Tai Chi involves synthesis — the means is the end. But the individual makes choices. A dancer can use Tai Chi, study it seriously and practice it diligently, and yet not be limited by it. Technically, an exciting performance involves risk. On the simplest physical level risk is absent from Tai Chi. You complete each shift of weight only after you have made sure of your new center. But a concert dancer who is always "careful" is too limited as a performer. Tai Chi focusses on process. With dancing the process is caught and distilled into performance.

Tai Chi is for the "long haul". Anyone with some time, good health and a little money can enjoy a few years, maybe many, of dancing; but Tai Chi will last the rest of your life, as long as you can find a small space and some time. It teaches survival and the peace that heals. Remember that lovely feeling, when you are ill, of waking from a soothing sleep? You can practice Tai Chi when you are feeling under the weather and sense that same restfulness as the body replenishes itself. Sometimes people find themselves "dreaming" Tai Chi. It begins to dance itself behind the eyes as you drift between sleep and waking, as comforting as being gently rocked to sleep.

It is within anybody's reach. No one is too awkward or too timid or too old. Everyone has a body — it is the one thing we share — and everyone is entitled to the discovery of that body and to the integration and health that discovery can bring.

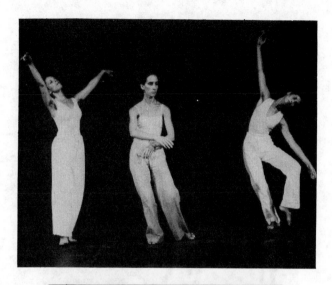

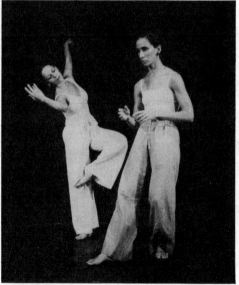

Playing Tai Chi the chest is pulled in softly, while the dancer's presence is outward-directed, and expansive. One can be used to balance the other. Tai Chi is rest and protection against injury for the hardworking dancer.

211

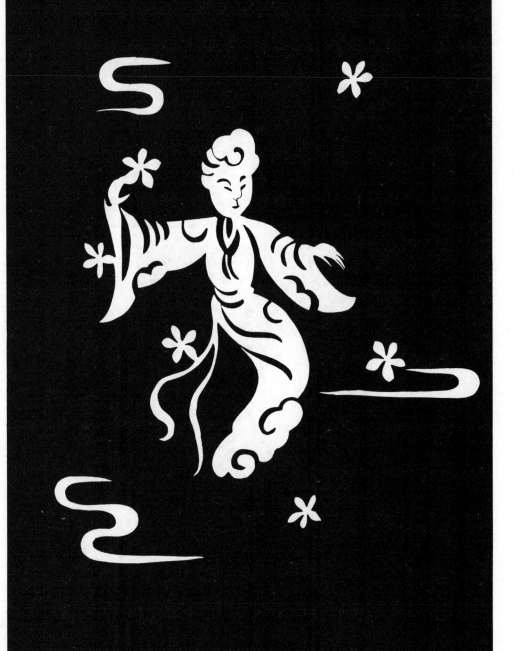

Tai Chi and Dance:
The Spontaneity of Form

This final essay is the result of several years of personal reflections, questions, and constant activity in and about the field of dance teaching and performance. The following discussions of dance are included in this book because dancers seem to me to suffer — in an especially heightened and visible form — the conflicts and frustrations endemic to all of us who are committed to a creative endeavor (define "creative" as broadly as you wish). And dance is the yang to Tai Chi's yin — the student of dance and the student of Tai Chi travel the same way.

S.K.

Consider the mirror and the possibility of reflection. A mirror that is clear and still reflects the world as it is.

213

Tai Chi Ch'uan

The agitated surface of a stormy body of water gives back a troubled image. Tai Chi is form through which to practice clarity of being; a way to still ourselves in order to see the world.

Spending a night fretting over a particularly difficult dilemma, I awaken with the despairing conviction that the tangle is inextricable. After an hour or two of Tai Chi practice, during which time the problem seems to be uselessly repeating itself inside my brain, I discover that somehow a decision has made itself. Shake a jar until all its different contents dissolve into murky confusion and then let it stand and watch the solutions settle out. You think a question to death until you finally give up, and the answer, or *an* answer, wells up from some unknown place. Sometimes it happens over the passage of time, years perhaps.

As you work, day by day, the same questions present themselves over and over. Through time, certain issues clarify and settle into patterns. The pattern is not an answer or a formula, but a constellation of questions, issues. Tai Chi is the study of the form and patterns of change, experienced by each of us in the life of the body and the spirit. The teachings of Tai Chi are characterized by a genuine simplicity. It stands as a useful metaphor for almost any process of integration, artistic or spiritual.

It is the perception of repetition that makes a work of art intelligible...

214

Tai Chi and Dance: The Spontaneity of Form

What each and every aesthetic object imposes upon us, in appropriate rhythms, is a unique and singular formula for the flow of our energy.

Bayer quoted by Susan Sontag

The time that is so fragmented as we live it appears in retrospect to have been a single, continuing search. Tai Chi begins with the obvious. And is always beginning again.

TO TEACH

Again and again with each class and rehearsal we ask ourselves just what it means — to teach, and to dance, and to teach dance. The talent of teaching is a separate and special gift, not the same as dancing itself. In the general category of learning experiences, the dance class is an odd subspecies. Students learn by physical imitation of the teacher, as much as from verbal images. Each class, from beginning to end, is (or should be) one integrated experience of movement. It is tempting, as a teacher, to force that experience through excessive use of your own energy, especially with beginning dancers who have little sense of how to sustain or project their own energy. This is the cheer-leading style of dance teaching; it is often successful, or at least popular, but it leaves the teacher drained and hoarse. "This is putting

215

out fire with fire, adding water to a flood; it is called adding to the excess" (Chuang Tzu). The teacher appears to be giving a great deal, but sometimes she is giving so much that the student is cheated of the chance to dance. The teacher who knows what she is doing creates with each class a progression of empty forms which the student is gently led to fill with her own flow of energy and motion.

Each student grows into a singular shape. Sometimes the way of working is reversal; other times the clichés demand to be worked through before you can emerge on the other side. A teacher senses when to work "against the grain", and provides problems in forms that lead the student into what does *not* come easily. Choreographically also, the material which comes easily in each individual case is often over-developed. ". . . the reversal of one's being means enlargement" (Jung). You can compose by elaboration as well as by refinement. No "way" is necessarily always more legitimate than all others.

A good teacher is not good for everyone, for each student's need of learning is different, and changes over time. The student needs to be supported, but also needs to know that there is someplace to go. In Mr. Lui's Tai Chi class, after he demonstrates a point or makes a correction, he watches the class try it a few times, smiling and silently nodding. What is there to say? We are learning that the means is the end. Tai Chi is always growing, so the practice becomes the pleasure.

In some Tai Chi classes the advanced students share a curiously erratic rhythm. This happens when the students, over a long period of time, mimic the teacher so diligently that they never discover their own rhythms. They copy the rise and fall of the teacher's form, from the outside. But the energy that creates the pattern is within, and can never be copied, only discovered. Think of the infinite possibilities of a snowflake. Resemblance pre-supposes distinction, on some level of perception. Artists hover jealously over their ideas, and complain loud and long about "rip-offs". An idea is no one's property. The energy of the original impulses, coherence, integrity of form — these can never be imitated. Mr. Lui tells us that if he gives away the ten secrets he knows today, he will surely know more tomorrow.

The most experienced and talented movement teachers I have known incorporated into their classes the whole of the Tai Chi circle, with its careful blending of opposites. Learning to teach, teaching to learn. The search is for that delicate balance, and the form that releases freedom. It is a constant struggle to vanquish the distractions of tension and the worry about "success", and to be able to center the whole self in the moment and focus on the rhythm of this class, these people, and their needs.

Modern dancers have often been uncomfortable with the distinction between improvisation and technique. They are both considered to be "merely" the means to an end. Technique, precise and careful information about the body, is passed on from teacher to teacher. Although it is not often formally codified, the fashions of the day rigidify very quickly. Improvisation, or the spontaneous creation of form, is a way out.

Every way out, of course, conceals its own trap. Technique too often loses its life and freshness, and yet the answer is not to substitute self-indulgence. Without labor there is no birth. In dance the technical aspect threatens to overwhelm the student, just because it is so difficult. But technique *serves* expression, or else it dies. In striving to execute more and more perfectly the given movements, the expressive source of motion is too often lost. Generations of dancers work to mold themselves into a pre-established style; but most techniques get their life from the authenticity of the work for which they are created. Imitated, technique is empty, reduced to gymnastic tricks. Eventually there are those who grow weary of the strenuous imitation. They proclaim once again the value of spontaneity — we will sit on stage and wiggle our toes, if we want to. If you think that's boring to watch, but you're afraid to say so because it is called "art", well, I agree with you. The pendulum swings to the other side, but either extreme is incomplete, by itself.

Good teaching must be concerned with the student dancer as more than a skilled automaton. Teaching a good class is more than the presentation and repetition of a series of pre-selected sequences. It requires the ability to focus on a particular quality or element of movement and follow it through, going further each time, beyond what you know or have done before. A careful plan is only a burden if you are never willing to be distracted from it by the exigencies of the moment. Each class is unexpected; each time you must locate again the channel of energy and follow faithfully, honestly, from the inside out. The problem is to allow an organic order to create itself, building from the solid base of a physical competence.

TO PERFORM

Modern dance as a performing art has grown now past the childhood of its first unselfconscious exuberance to a more introspective stage. (adolescence?) It has turned inward, focussing on the nature and mechanics of performance itself. The form of the art has become its own subject matter, like some mythical creature consuming itself. I am not talking now so much about major modern and ballet companies which for the most part still treat performance as a kind of spectacle, but of a growing movement originating with the Judson Church in the 60s and expanding in ever-widening circles from there. (For an excellent summary of the history of modern dance see the chapter "Modern Dance" by Jill Johnston in *The New*

American.) Very broadly speaking the development up through Cunningham was from the narrative form of traditional ballet, through a more abstract but still dramatic style of "modern" dance, to Merce Cunningham's random and uninflected composition of clear, spare, classical movement. Cunningham exemplifies an extreme reaction to the traditional concern with narrative and dramatic form. The extent to which his heresies have become dogma is a measure of his undisputed genius. But dogma *is* dogmatic, and we forget easily that it is one man's personal contribution to a long and developing history. Cunningham has answered the question in one way — using variations on chance procedure as a composing mechanism. It is also a liberation from the habitual; a path to the unfamiliar. Brilliant perhaps, but hardly the last word on the subject. There cannot be a "last word" if our commitment is to authentic change and not to mere hero worship.

In the years since the sixties, the alleged avant-garde has dealt, more and less honestly, with the familiar questions of style. New developments began with the Happenings — previously distinct media began to be integrated and the focus was on spontaneity of form. Today there are quite a few young and genuinely original choreographers, most of them working independently, or with a few other dancers. Current works of interest vary widely in form, conception, and stylistic choices. The ideas of the current group of performers as they parallel those of other kinds of modern artists, have been well and elegantly articulated. The point of view is as appealing as it is ambivalent. Self-justification is also a kind of art — why not?

> The notions of silence, emptiness and reduction stretch out new prescriptions for looking, hearing, etc. . . . furnished with impoverished art, purged by silence, one might then be able to begin to transcend the frustrating selectivity of attention . . . Ideally one should be able to pay attention to everything.
>
> Susan Sontag, *Styles of Radical Will*,
> "The Aesthetics of Silence"

If form is everywhere, then the function of the artist can be to focus our attention — on the Campbell soup can, as well as on anything else. Through a kind of austerity and deliberate inexpressiveness, we are led to pay attention to the small as well as the great; we are led to the rediscovery of the silence in the midst of things.

Lao Tzu would undoubtedly approve of the theory. Unfortunately, the theory is more appealing than the work, a reversal of the usual case, where the criticism pales beside the art. The performances are too often *merely* conceptual, leaving a flat and empty feeling. The most positive reaction is a grudging recognition of the artist's "cleverness". Is it because the work expresses the emptiness of life? Does it have to be boring to be about boredom? Or is it a new version of the old story of the emperor's new clothes. The art is *so* conceptual that you must be initiated to appreciate it. It creates a closed elite of sophisticated viewers, jaded, and hipper-than-thou. And any word of criticism automatically dismisses the critic as "merely" old-fashioned.

Each artist seems to be involved in a fruitless search to do something that has never been done before. Everything has been said; we are deafened by the monotonous drone of all the words, pictures, and melodies of the past. What next but silence? It is a position with an undeniable intellectual integrity; but art, and performance especially, is not solely an intellectual activity.

In the course of time each thing gives birth to its opposite. Growth includes the integration of the one with the other, not the destruction of one by the other. Brutally tearing up the roots of the past creates an empty, violent art, when we need genuine nourishment. "The efficacious artwork leaves silence in its wake" (Sontag). After a film, or book, or play, there is that moment of emptiness; the space surrounding the form. But it does not then follow that silence itself is a substitute for the work, except by a kind of double-talk. Real silence reverberates with echoes. Silence without sound is not different from sound without silence.

Let's say I invite you to my theatre for a "performance", and this piece is a half-hour of nothing. No movement, no sound, nothing. For that half-hour, you sit with your own thoughts, and your expectations. Perhaps you become aware of the quality of the light in the room, or the sounds on the street outside. The emptiness of the work is a focus for your attention on yourself and the world around you, for that time, in that place. Perhaps you will enjoy it, if you are sympathetic towards me, or particularly open-minded. But is it really any more than an interesting exercise? What is the balancing point at which substance and thought are woven together?

It is often said that the ideal way to come to the experience of a work of art is without any expectations, that is, empty. Everyone admits by now that this is not completely possible. At the very least, *I* have one expectation — to be touched. I want to witness and share in someone's (the artist's) struggle to give form to something "cared about". It isn't that art must be representational, either. Clever exercises in design and conception leave me cold. But abstract images can be delicately suggestive. Space and line and the punctuation of time can touch us, even if we cannot articulate an "interpretation".

At its best art teaches us openness to all experience. It does not follow though, that all experience is the same, or that we are affected by everything in the same way, that is to say, not at all. Existentialism can be reduced to romantic affectation.

Dancing is perhaps the most demanding of all the performing arts. It requires not only the most refined, strenuous and daily use of the total physical being, but also the most extreme psychological vulnerability. The performer is completely visible, seen in a way that most of us are seen only by intimate friends and lovers. There is no distance in the medium — the work is inseparable from the actual physical presence of the dancer. It is this that can make the dancer such an insane mixture of vanity and self-abnegation. (Like Tai Chi, dancing is a good model of "being-present-in-the-moment". In class or rehearsal, if you attempt a difficult step and fail, you try again. You are forced to let go of your failures; if you hold onto the frustrations of each attempt, paralysis sets in. You learn a kind of patience with yourself — each time is new.)

Each performance is unique — the work is created over and over again. In the case of pre-set or choreographed pieces (which most modern dance and all ballet has been until relatively recently) the dancer repeats the same sequence of movements thousands of times in rehearsal and performance. And yet if it is to work, it must be rediscovered each time. The "form" of Tai Chi is a model of this kind of "spontaneous repetition". And in the case of dance-works structured improvisationally, the dance is literally created anew with each performance and rehearsal. This is perhaps the ultimate in "presentness", in the unity of form and formlessness. Good improvisation is *not* formless; it is precisely and exquisitely formed, as it happens. It is very, very rare.

The dialectic continues between composition and

improvisation. Images must be clarified without being eviscerated. The dancer must cultivate an instinctive and absolutely honest responsiveness. This is a precious gift in these times, and a life-sustaining one. In an effort to survive the daily onslaught of horror we have systematically extinguished our sensibility. Otherwise who could read the first few pages of any morning newspaper without drowning in tears? As a tactic of survival, it backfires as we become more and more brittle. We lose our resilience, and are ever more liable to break, one morning or afternoon, with an unexpected and irreversible snap.

Unlike dance performances, works of painting, music, and literature are preserved by their very nature. Traditionally at least this is true, although since the Happenings the visual arts have been encroaching on the natural province of performance. Even a play, which comes alive in performance, is still expressive on the page. Dances can be notated, it is true, but the system is laborious and cumbersome and results in a record, not a re-creation. Of course the techniques of video and film have made it possible to preserve and re-create dance electronically, but this is a function of the recording medium and not of dance itself.

It has often happened that painters and writers, considered to be failures in their life-times, have been judged differently by "history". This is never possible for a dancer, or indeed for any performer — the performer lives and works inside the moment. There is no

225

before and no after. Perhaps this is why works of dance seem to "date" so quickly. Twenty or thirty years later a particular style of dancing reproduced with slavish accuracy is usually no more than an historical curiosity.

All of this makes the issue of critical response and judgment painfully ambiguous. On the one hand the dancer is freed of the confines of history, since the work exists only while it is being done. At the same time the dancer is the absolute prisoner of time. There is no recourse, no court of appeal. There is only the judgment of your contemporaries, bound as they are by the passing moods of fashion and prejudice. Add to this the intense and involuted nature of the world of professional dance. The conflicts and vanities of ego take their toll.

You are always performing *for* somebody, there is always the unavoidable question of response and popularity. For the performer the battle is often pitched between integrity and accessibility. But you could hardly say that the lines are clearly drawn. And of course there is money. To work you must eat; to win grants you must be judged to be "successful".

In dancing more than any other art, the source is the self. Begin where you are — "A journey of a thousand miles starts from beneath one's feet" (Lao Tzu, of course). One unfortunate and uncomfortable modern tangent is the confusion of theatre with therapy. Probably the less said about that the better. Unhappily, the serious and honest young dancer-choreographer can easily become

226

trapped here, at this hopefully fertile beginning. The work turns inward; you are soon suffocated by your own familiarity with yourself. Or there is the opposite pitfall of constant self-dramatization. Television culture has made models of performers without material, celebrities who play one role — themselves.

Life is interchange between the self and the world — the channels must be open, and to be open they must be empty. In order to let the self out, learn to let the world in. If perception is unremittingly turned inward, no matter how honorable the intention, the work cannot grow, and must be stale and insipid. We are too quick to lower our voices reverently at the mention of art. "I'm only a craftsman — how would I have any art?" To be a workman, that's what Chuang Tzu counsels — to value workmanship.

To continue the litany of contradictions, if you are a performer, dancing your work, you can never see it. You can experience it from the inside, but beyond that you are dependent on the response of your audience. But any audience is a collection of conflicting sensibilities. Integrity and coherence are short-lived if you begin to substitute the judgment of others for your own. On the other hand, to go on you must be able to doubt what you have done. Progress is not always, or necessarily, towards success. And so we resign ourselves happily to perpetual angst. We never desire what is present, but only what is inaccessible. By concentrating on the incomplete we assure ourselves of a permanent sense of loss. Wanting gives us more pleasure than having. Our imaginations are graceful in direct proportion to the ill-concealed desperation of our lives.

IN THE END

In the course of this book we've found ourselves repeating one thing many times, and in many ways — to a Western sensibility Oriental thought appears temptingly, deceptively, simple. We fool ourselves if we pretend that we can be children once again, or think that we can assume at will the impassive serenity of a picture-book Buddha. Certain kinds of cultural wishfulness are doomed to failure. No matter how appealing, the manners and mores of another time and place cannot be acquired like fashionable antique clothing. Cultural roots lie beyond our reach, in unconscious depths.

Or do they? The world grows smaller day by day. And in our time, this "age of anthropology", the walls between cultures are crumbling fast. Many people are struggling to create new cultural modes out of the bits and pieces. There are more and more questions to which the answers are not automatically given. Cultural imperatives are less clear; economic imperatives are less clear. At least for the middle class, conscious choice is more and more the deciding factor in "life style" decisions.

Our cup is half-empty. Oriental wisdom sees the cup as half-full. There *are* contradictions and difficult questions to resolve. There is the issue of the cultivation of the inner self at the expense of the social conscience. Some ideas have a kind of neutrality that makes them prey to every passing partisan cause. With respect to Eastern philosophy one problem is perspective. Can you excuse political and social inaction on the grounds of a grand and cosmic view of things? The "path" leads to a place of peace, where the rumbling of the troubled world is a distant murmur. But there is no excuse for resignation, or the deliberate ignorance of a privileged class. Looking beyond our time, can we still live inside it with integrity? What you see depends on where you stand, and in which direction you turn your eyes. Can you choose to be conscious only of the "great circle" which, changing forever, never changes? Don't you have to act from where *you* stand? Do we admit a moral obligation to be true to our own time and place? Will we escape from the prisons of our expectations? In choosing for ourselves must we judge one another, and threaten one another? You can never see through my eyes — but what do we see when we look together? If we begin in the same circle, we will surely meet, no matter which way we go.

The methods of the East teach submission to "natural law" through ease and relaxation. There are other legitimate paths to liberation. What about the taking of risks? Learning through recklessness? The violent de-

229

-struction of earthquake and flood is as "natural" as the gentle change of the seasons. From the East we might learn how to see death as change and so to make our uneasy peace with it. We congratulate ourselves on our scientific discoveries and the fact that we no longer die of bubonic plague. Is it better to die of some bizarre new industrial cancer? When my grandfather died, peacefully, I couldn't be with him because hospital rules forbid children. Yet violent death, of every conceivable variety, is accessible to a child at the flip of a television switch. In spite of us, the circle will complete itself. Thinking to defeat death, we have only changed the specifics.

The struggle for survival — we all know what it means, even if we are lucky enough never to have had to fight for our literal survival. It is no easy task — to survive with generosity, to go in peace. And yet in some way, we *can* choose the style of our struggle, we *can* shape the quality of our energy. East and West look at one another and learn. Looking towards the other, we see ourselves, or some way that we would like to be.

A recommendation.

A wider realm of possibility.

Other Books on Tai Chi Ch'uan

This is a selective listing which includes only books which we feel we can recommend.

T'ai Chi Ch'uan for Health and Self-Defense by T. T. Liang, Redwing Book Company, Boston, 1974. A short, inexpensive paperback. Good explanations of The Classics and a sound exposition of Tai Chi.

T'ai-Chi: The "Supreme Ultimate" Exercise for Health, Sport, and Self-Defense by Cheng Man-ch'ing and Robert Smith, Charles Tuttle, Rutland, Vermont, 1967. This book has a very short text and extensive photographs of Cheng Man-ching performing Tai Chi and Push Hands. The book is expensive, but useful for more advanced and serious students because of the photos.

Lee's Modified Tai Chi for Health by Lee Ying-arng, Unicorn Press, Hong Kong, 1968. Once you get past the five prefaces, two forwards, and the introduction this book contains a lot of information about Tai Chi including interesting photos of some of the old masters. Lee himself seems to be rather enterprising, offering a Correspondence Course complete with a certificate, a guarantee, and an 8 mm. film.

Tai Chi Chuan: A Simplified Method of Calisthentics by Cheng Man-ch'ing, Shih Chung Tai-chi Chuan Center, Taiwan, 1962. This book is difficult to come by, but quite good, with a much longer text than the book written by the author in conjunction with Robert Smith.

Embrace Tiger, Return to Mountain — the Essence of T'ai Chi, by Al Chung-liang Huang, Real People Press, Moab, Utah, 1973. This book represents one extreme of Tai Chi, the undisciplined, free-form style. The book, however, is quite interesting, with some good exercises and a useful perspective on Tai Chi and the spirit which it embodies. The book is saved for me by the fact that Mr. Huang can occasionally laugh at himself.

T'ai Chi Ch'uan: Its Effects and Practical Applications by Yearning K. Chen, Unicorn Press, Hong Kong, 1971.

T'ai Chi Ch'uan by Sophia Delza, Cornerstone Library, New York, 1961. Slightly dated.

Tai Chi for Health by Edward Maisel, Dell, New York, 1963.

Fundamentals of Tai Chi Ch'uan by We-Shan Huang, South Sky Book Company, Hong Kong, 1973. Long and extensive, written by a man with wonderful credentials, but incomprehensible to us in English.

Books of Related Interest from

CHICAGO REVIEW PRESS

SPRING & ASURA — Poems of Kenji Miyazawa   Cloth **$6.50**
Translated by Hiroaki Sato   Paperback **$3.50**
Introduction by Burton Watson

"Not only perhaps the foremost Japanese poet since Basho and Buson, but a cranky humble world stature poet . . . A book we Americans both need & will vastly enjoy has been given us."

— *Gary Snyder*

"An important addition to representative collections of world poetry."

— *Library Journal*

POEMS OF A PENISIST — Mutsuo Takahashi   Cloth **$10.00**
Translated by Hiroaki Sato   Paperback **$4.95**
Introduction by Burton Watson

"Like his fellow countryman, Yukio Mishima, Mutsuo Takahashi transmutes violence-tinged erotic love of young men into high art. The touching "Christ for thieves" alone makes the volume worth purchasing for collections concerned with the interaction of East and West in literature or homosexuality."
— *Choice*

"Mr. Hiroaki Sato, to whom we are also grateful for a magnificent Kenji Miyazawa, is beyond praise: a translator of genius . . ."
— *Journal of the Association of Teachers of Japanese*

THE SILVER SPOON by Naka Kansuke   Cloth **$10.00**
Translated and with   Paperback **$4.95**
an introduction by Etsuko Terasaki

A modern Japanese classic, *The Silver Spoon* is an extraordinary evocation of childhood and a memoir of the daily life, customs, folk manners, and the children's games of pre-World War I Japan. This translation makes *The Silver Spoon* available in English for the first time.